The Profession of Dietetics

A Team Approach

The Profession of Dietetics

A Team Approach

Second Edition

June Payne-Palacio
Pepperdine University

Deborah D. Canter
Kansas State University

Prentice Hall
Upper Saddle River, New Jersey   *Columbus, Ohio*

Library of Congress Cataloging-in-Publication Data

Payne-Palacio, June

    The profession of dietetics : a team approach / June Payne-Palacio, Deborah D. Canter.—2nd ed.

      p. cm.

    Includes bibliographical references and index.

    ISBN 0-13-646886-1

    1. Dietetics—Vocational guidance.   I. Canter, Deborah D. II. Title.

    RM218.5.P39   2000

613.2—dc21   99-32799

                                                            CIP

Editor: Neil W. Marquardt
Editorial Assistant: Susan Kegler
Production Editor: Linda Hillis Bayma
Copy Editor: Luanne Dreyer Elliott
Design Coordinator: Diane C. Lorenzo
Text Designer: STELLARViSIONs
Cover Designer: Diane C. Lorenzo
Production Manager: Laura Messerly
Electronic Text Management: Marilyn Wilson Phelps, Karen L. Bretz,
    Melanie N. King
Illustrations: Colin Hayes
Marketing Manager: Shannon M. Simonsen
Marketing Assistant: Adam Kloza

This book was set in Bookman and Futura by Prentice Hall and was printed and bound by R.R. Donnelley & Sons Company. The cover was printed by Phoenix Color Corp.

Photo credits: Photos on pp. 42 (top), 43, 44, 50, 52, and 102 provided by June Payne-Palacio.

Printed in the United States of America

10 9 8 7 6 5 4 3 2 1

ISBN: 0-13-646886-1

Prentice-Hall International (UK) Limited, *London*
Prentice-Hall of Australia Pty. Limited, *Sydney*
Prentice-Hall of Canada, Inc., *Toronto*
Prentice-Hall Hispanoamericana, S. A., *Mexico*
Prentice-Hall of India Private Limited, *New Delhi*
Prentice-Hall of Japan, Inc., *Tokyo*
Prentice-Hall (Singapore) Pte. Ltd., *Singapore*
Editora Prentice-Hall do Brasil, Ltda., *Rio de Janeiro*

Preface

This book is written for students interested in finding out more about the profession of dietetics. Understanding who dietetics professionals are, what dietetics professionals do, and how to become a dietary manager, dietetic technician, or registered dietitian is a complex task. Few other professions offer so many educational routes for entry or so many ways to practice one's trade. While this diversity is a strength, it often confuses those who wish to enter the profession, as well as prospective customers who are trying to understand who dietetics professionals are or why they should consult one.

It is the goal of this book to present a clear and up-to-date picture of the profession of dietetics and try to answer some basic questions:

- What is a profession, and how does dietetics qualify as a profession?
- How has the history of the profession shaped dietetics practice today?
- Who are members of the dietetics team, and how do they work together?
- What is The American Dietetic Association, and why should one become a member?
- What is credentialing of dietetics professionals, and why is it important?
- What kinds of positions are filled by dietetics professionals?
- What does the future hold for dietetics practice?

The profession of dietetics is dynamic, exciting, and in need of enthusiastic, energetic, and visionary men and women who wish to join the team. It is our hope that this book enlightens, informs, and inspires those who read it. If this occurs, then our dream for this book will have been achieved.

ACKNOWLEDGMENTS

The authors thank the following reviewers for their insightful suggestions: For the first edition, Rebecca L. Bradley, University of Alabama, Birmingham; Dorothy Pond-Smith, Washington State University; and Martha L. Taylor, University of North Carolina, Greensboro. For the second edition, Sara Long Anderson, Southern Illinois University, Carbondale; Gail Gates, Oklahoma State University; Lucy C. Robinson, Northern Illinois University; Anne M. Smith, The Ohio State University; and Martha L. Taylor, University of North Carolina, Greensboro.

Brief Contents

Contents

PART THREE   PREPARING FOR PRACTICE

PART FOUR   PROFESSIONAL ASSOCIATIONS

Chapter 6   Professionalism   101

Chapter 7   The American Dietetic Association   131

Chapter 8   The Dietary Managers Association   **149**

PART FIVE   THE FUTURE

Chapter 9   Trends and Predictions   **161**

Index   **171**

PART ONE

The Past

CHAPTER 1

A Brief History of Dietetics

ANCIENT HISTORY

The role of food in curing, preventing, or causing illness has been recognized since the beginning of recorded history. "If a man has pain inside, food and drink coming back to his mouth . . . let him refrain from eating onions for three days" is the first known written dietary recommendation, carved on Babylonian stone tablets about 2500 B.C.[1] The typical daily regimen during this time consisted of barley paste or bread, onions, a few beans, and beer. The Book of Judges in the Old Testament contains a prenatal dietary prescription that has withstood the test of time: "Therefore beware, and drink no wine or strong drink, and eat nothing unclean, for lo, you shall conceive and bear a son."[2]

The word *diet* is from the Greek *diaita* meaning "manner of living."[3] It appears in many early writings, including those of Hippocrates and Galen.[4] The oldest known cookbook, *Apicius*, (approximately 100 B.C.) contains many dietetic principles that are still sound today.[5] In ancient China, food therapy was practiced as a special branch of medicine.[6] Chinese observations about diabetes date to the third century,[7] and descriptions of night blindness and its correct dietary cure date to the seventh century.[8]

THE MIDDLE AGES

Hospital records from St. Bartholomew's Hospital, founded in Britain in 1123, provide the first written evidence of a typical hospital menu. Bread and beer formed the basis of the diet.[9] This obviously inadequate and unpalatable diet led to a prevalence of scurvy among patients. Other conditions in early British hospitals were also poor. Sanitation was nonexistent, there was overcrowding, buildings were unsafe, and stern disciplinary measures were used on noncompliant patients.

With the publication of *De re Medicina* in 1478 in Florence, diet became an important part of medical practice. In this publication, medicine was divided into three branches—diseases treated manually, diseases treated by medicine, and diseases treated by diet. In 1480, the first printed cookbook appeared, containing reference to quality and varieties of meat, fish, fruits, and vegetables, how they nourish the body, and how they should be prepared.[10]

PROGRESS IN THE EIGHTEENTH AND NINETEENTH CENTURIES

Until the eighteenth century, beliefs and writings about diet were based on insufficient scientific evidence. But with advances in chemistry and physics came the foundation necessary to establish dietetics as a profession. Lavoisier's work on digestion is generally regarded as the first modern, scientific research on nutrition.[11]

Still, progress was slow. A patient in an English hospital in the eighteenth century would receive the only menu served:

Four to five ounces of meat (usually already boiled for the broth)

Three-quarters to one pound of bread

Two to three pints of beer

Pottage or pudding

Fruits and vegetables were missing from this daily allowance—they were suspected by some as being harmful and by others as having medicinal, rather than nutritive value. Small amounts of cheese, butter, roots, and greens were sometimes included in the daily fare. Family and friends could bring food to supplement the meager hospital offerings, or patients could buy food from the food sellers who came through the wards.

The most expensive item on the menu was the beer. Doctors of the time believed that alcohol was necessary to treat illness. Since water was contaminated, beer was used extensively. When cost-cutting measures were instituted, the beer allowance was reduced or completely eliminated.

Patients who were unable to eat the full diet or complained about the food were disciplined. Punishments included cutting the food allowance in half, omitting some meals entirely, or restricting patients to toast and water for a week.[12]

In American hospitals too, food was given little thought and conditions were very poor. The first hospitals in the United States were in Philadelphia—Philadelphia General Hospital was built in 1731, and Pennsylvania Hospital was built in 1751.[13] Mush and molasses was the usual fare, with a pint of beer included for supper.[14] After the War of 1812, fruit was added to the menu as a garnish.

There was little improvement in hospital conditions until the humanitarian movement of the late nineteenth century. Great progress was made between 1850 and 1920.

Florence Nightingale (1820–1910), a superintendent of nurses in British military hospitals in Turkey during the Crimean War (1854–1856), established foodservice for the troops (Figure 1.1). With the help of a French chef, Alexis Soyer, she reduced the death rate of injured soldiers by improving diet and sanitary conditions. Later, in her writings and nursing practice, Nightingale continued to demonstrate her belief in the importance of nutrition and foodservice management by emphasizing the selection and service of food and the art and science of feeding the sick.[15]

Sarah Tyson Rorer (1849–1937) is considered to be the first American dietitian (Figure 1.2). Her training consisted of some medical school lectures and a three-month cooking course. In 1878, Sarah Rorer opened the Philadelphia Cooking School, where students learned about food values, protein, and carbohydrates, but nothing about calories and vitamins. Students took ten classes in chemistry, several on

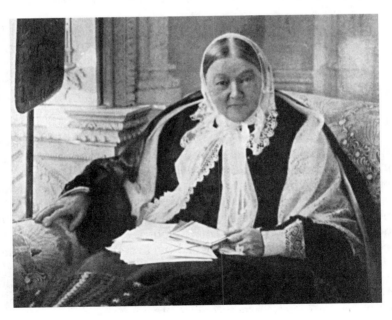

Figure 1.1
Florence Nightingale.

Source: Courtesy of the Florence Nightingale Museum, London.

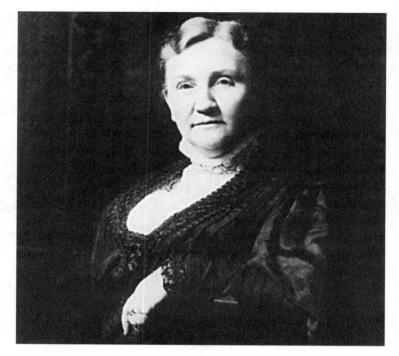

Figure 1.2
Sarah Tyson Rorer.

Source: Photo courtesy of The American Dietetic Association.

physiology and hygiene, and ten classes on cooking for the sick. Twelve students graduated each year for 33 years, and they secured positions planning meals and supervising production in hospital kitchens.[16]

In 1877, the American Medical Association formed a Committee on Dietetics and asked Rorer to edit a new publication entitled *The Dietetic Gazette*.[17] Later, she published *Household News* on her own, in which she wrote articles on topics such as feeding the sick and designing a kitchen and answered questions regarding diet from readers.[18] In her lifetime, she wrote more than fifty books and booklets and wrote articles for such magazines as *Ladies' Home Journal*, *Table Talk*, and *Good Housekeeping*.[19] Rorer also established the first diet kitchen and dietary counseling service, at the request of three well-known physicians.

In 1896, the U.S. Department of Agriculture (USDA) published *Bulletin 28*, the first food composition tables.[20] It was an indispensable resource for dietetic practitioners for many years.

At the Lake Placid Conference on Home Economics in 1899, the term *dietitian* was first defined. The conference attendees determined that the title *dietitian* should be "applied to persons who specialize in the knowledge of food and can meet the demands of the medical profession for diet therapy."[21]

THE YOUNG PROFESSION IN THE TWENTIETH CENTURY

The Iowa Agricultural School in Ames was probably the first college to offer courses in cookery, in 1872. A yearly course in "household chemistry," which included cookery, was begun in 1877 at the Kansas State Agricultural College in Manhattan.[22] Other colleges and universities soon followed their lead. The first internship for dietitians was established by Florence Corbett in 1903, at the New York Department of Charities. Applicants for the three-month course had to be over 25 years of age, have taught for one year, and be domestic science graduates.

At about the same time, Casimir Funk discovered a chemical substance named *amine*. Since this substance appeared essential to life, he added the prefix *vita*.[23] Discovery of the individual "vitamines" would come much later, but this initial discovery was a milepost in nutritional history.

In 1910, dietitians were practicing in poorly defined roles with a diversity of titles, but they were facing some of the same problems that dietitians face today. Few people could define the role of the dietist, dietician, dietitian, or nutrition worker, as dietitians were variously called. The title *nutritionist* appeared in the early 1920s, and the spelling *dietitian* was agreed upon in 1930.[24]

Fighting faddism and quackery was an issue in 1910, just as it is today. Fletcherizing, or chewing each mouthful of food 32 times before swallowing, is an example of a harmless but ineffective popular notion of that day. Calorie counting, high-protein or low-protein diets, and natural foods were other popular fads.

Nutritional research received an unexpected boost in importance with the outbreak of World War I. The examination of 2.5 million military draftees in Great Britain in 1917 found 41 percent to be in poor health and unfit for military duty, due most commonly to nutritional status.[25] In the United States, the American Red Cross enrolled dietitians for army duty. In World War I, 356 dietitians served in the armed services. Mary de Garmo Bryan, who later became the second president of The American Dietetic Association, was among them (Figures 1.3 through 1.5). The nutritional expertise of these brave dietitians provided leadership for both the nourishment of hospitalized soldiers and the general public at home. Conservation of food was encouraged, as dietitians advised the government on efficient methods of food production, distribution, and preparation (Figure 1.6).

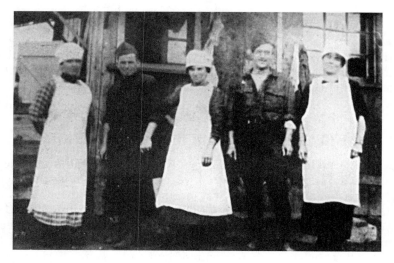

Figure 1.3
Mary de Garmo Bryan and a field kitchen staff during
World War I.

Source: Photo courtesy of The American Dietetic Association.

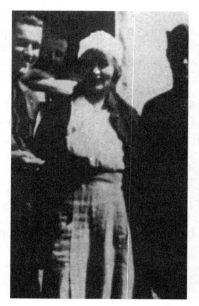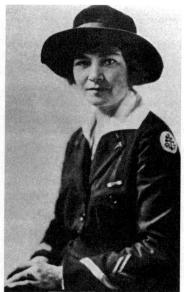

Figure 1.4
Dietitians' Red Cross uniforms from World War I: *left,* a
duty uniform of blue crepe with Red Cross cape and
right, a gray travel uniform.

Source: Photos courtesy of The American Dietetic Association.

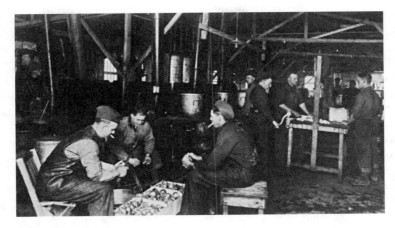

Figure 1.5
General kitchen and mess hall, Savenay, France, 1919.

Source: Photo courtesy of The American Dietetic Association.

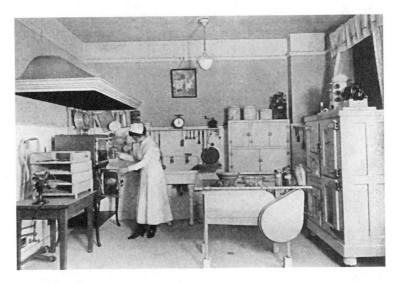

Figure 1.6
Mary E. Pascoe, dietitian for the New York Edison Company (now Consolidated Edison), demonstrating the correct method for drying food in an electric oven in 1917. Note utensils of the period and one of the first domestic refrigerators.

Source: Courtesy of the Consolidated Edison Co. of New York, Inc.

When the American Home Economic Association decided not to hold its annual meeting in 1917 because of the war, two dietitians, Lenna Frances Cooper and Lulu G. Graves, organized a special meeting of hospital dietitians to discuss emergency war needs. Out of this meeting of 98 people, The American Dietetic Association (ADA) was formed. This association, with 39 charter members and dues of $1 per year, was formed to address the interests of dietitians. Its first president was Lulu Graves (Figure 1.7), who was head of the dietary department at Lakeside Hospital in Cleveland (Figure 1.8). The first meeting of ADA was held in the basement at Lakeside Hospital. Graves

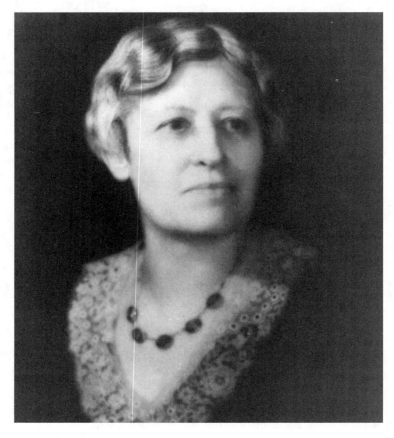

Figure 1.7
Lulu Graves

Source: Photo courtesy of The American Dietetic Association.

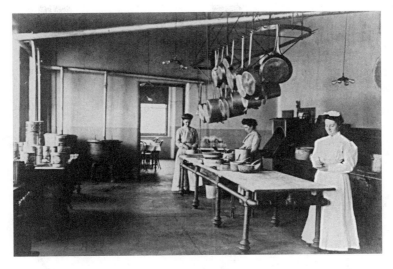

Figure 1.8
Lakeside Hospital kitchen, 1905. The first meeting of The
American Dietetic Association was held here in 1917.

Source: Photo courtesy of University Hospitals, Cleveland.

served as president for the first three years. Lenna Frances Cooper
(Figure 1.9) served as first vice president. The continuing history of
ADA will be covered in Chapter 7 and the history of education of
dietetic practitioners, in Chapter 4.

Dieto-therapy as practiced in the early 1900s consisted of many
special diets like the Sippy Diet for ulcers, which consisted of cream
and poached eggs. Diabetic diets varied widely even after the discovery
of insulin in 1921.

The passage of the federal Maternity and Infancy Act in the 1920s
allowed state health departments to employ nutritionists.[26] The passage of Title V of the Social Security Act in 1935 provided major
impetus for the employment of nutrition consultants in state and
local health departments by making federal funds available for this
purpose.[27]

The profession of dietetics continued to become more widely recognized and broaden in scope. World War II contributed to the public
recognition of the role of dietitians: Nearly 2,000 dietitians were com-
missioned in the armed services, while many others educated the public at home (Figures 1.10 and 1.11). The practice of dietetics broadened
to include institutions such as restaurants, airlines, and industrial

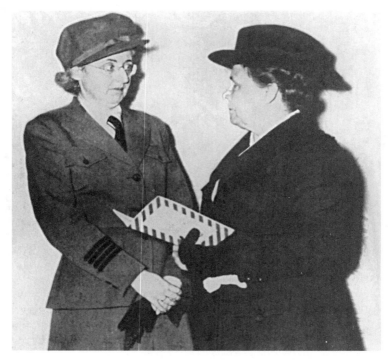

Figure 1.9
Lenna Frances Cooper (left) in a World War I uniform and
Helen Burns (right) in a World War II uniform at the twenty-
fifth anniversary of The American Dietetic Association in
1942.

Source: Photo courtesy of The American Dietetic Association.

plants. After the war, dietitians were granted full military status and
their position in the healthcare setting strengthened with the emphasis
on allied health professions and the healthcare team concept.[28]

Passage of the National School Lunch Act in 1946 expanded dietetics to include the establishment of school lunch programs, including
the training of personnel in foodservice and nutrition education. The
Hill–Burton Hospital Facilities Survey and Construction Act (1946)
and the Medicare and Medicaid legislation of the 1960s created
demand for the services of consultant dietitians in healthcare facilities
such as nursing homes. The civil rights movement of the 1960s
brought the issues of poverty and hunger into the political spotlight.

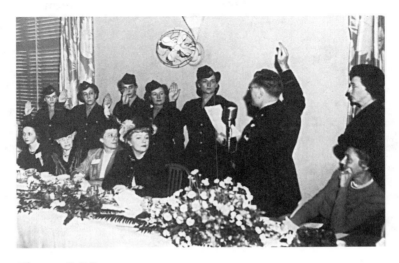

Figure 1.10
Army dietitians receive permanent rank, 1947.

Source: Photo courtesy of The American Dietetic Association.

The government instituted its war on poverty, and Senator Hubert Humphrey worked with the Senate Select Committee on Nutrition and Human Needs.[29] As a result of these and other efforts, the USDA food assistance programs to low-income families were established or expanded in the 1970s. Important among these were the food stamp program and school lunch and breakfast programs; child care and summer foodservice for children; supplemental feeding programs for women, infants, and children (WIC); and nutrition for the elderly.[30]

Food assistance programs have developed more rapidly and with more support than nutrition education programs. In 1968, the Cooperative Extension Service of the USDA began the Expanded Food and Nutrition Education Program (EFNEP), which provides nutrition and food education for low-income families. In 1975, three years after the start of the WIC program, an education component was legislated. And, in 1977, nutrition education was incorporated into the food stamp program. The Food And Agriculture Act of 1977 included the Nutrition Education and Training Program (NETP or NET), the first federal nutrition program for children.[31] The ADA and others express the need for making nutrition education a primary component of *all* food assistance programs.[32]

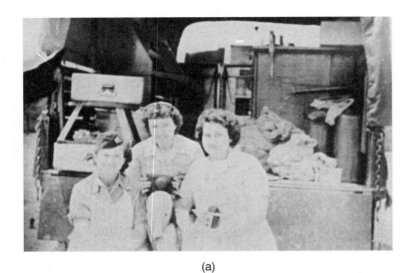

(a)

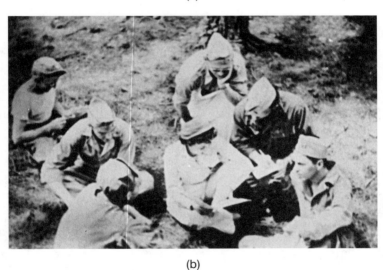

(b)

Figure 1.11
Equipment changes in a field kitchen in World War II, but dietitians teach anytime and anywhere.

Source: Photos courtesy of The American Dietetic Association.

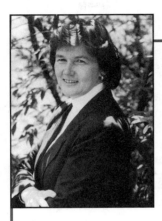

PROFILE

Jo Anne Cassell, M.S., R.D.

POSITION
   Author/editor/nutrition consultant in private
      practice
EDUCATION
   B.S. University of Oklahoma, Norman, OK
   M.S. in Nutrition, Texas Woman's University,
      Denton, TX
   Pursuing Ph.D. in Nutrition, Texas Woman's
      University, Denton, TX. Anticipated date of
      completion, August 2000.
ROUTE TO REGISTRATION
   Graduate assistantship

◆ **Professional Involvement**
   Although I joined the ADA as soon as I was qualified to do so, my
   involvement was minimal for a number of years. I took advantage of
   the benefits of membership but felt little responsibility to contribute. A
   turning point came in 1982, when I was hired as the research associate
   for the 1984 Study Commission on Dietetics. That position drew me
   into close contact with the distinguished seven-member panel
   appointed to the Commission but also to the ADA professional staff,
   elected and appointed leadership of the Association, and outstanding
   dietetic practitioners across the nation. For 18 months Commission
   members looked at all aspects of the profession and the Association. It
   was their task to look at the past and the present and then make recommendations for the future. It was my task to assist them in that work
   and to write the background papers and drafts of each recommendation. Those conclusions and recommendations were published in 1984
   as *A New Look at the Profession of Dietetics*. The work left me with a
   new respect for the men and women who have given so generously of
   their time and energy over the years to provide leadership for the Association. And, I found an even greater respect for the role played by the
   Association in helping to improve the health of Americans and influencing public policy on nutrition-related issues.
   I was hired by the ADA Foundation to write a history of the Association entitled *Carry the Flame: A History of The American Dietetic Association*. There can be no better way to learn about a person, profession,
   or association than to delve so thoroughly into history. I also learned
   that preparing a history opens doors to the future. You can hardly learn

about history without failing to see trends, themes, and cycles that have implications for the future.

For six years I was the editor of a professional journal of dietetics, *Topics in Clinical Nutrition*. That experience provided continual insight into current research in dietetics, as well as an excellent introduction to outstanding dietetics practitioners across the nation.

In the 1990s, because of my long involvement with the development of the Fellow and Specialty Credentialing programs with the Commission on Dietetic Registration, I was asked to serve on the Steering Committees of three separate role delineation studies. Those experiences gave me a focused look at exactly what dietetics practitioners were doing today in their work settings.

These unique opportunities have made me a strong advocate for the profession of dietetics. They have left me with a great respect for past and present leadership in the Association and great confidence in the capable new leadership now emerging to meet the changing circumstances in healthcare. I see dietitians trained in new ways to meet those changing circumstances, and I envy them the exciting years ahead.

◆ **Words of Wisdom for Future Dietetics Professionals**
Remember that your training has given you a solid foundation for beginning your new career. But also remember that if you don't continue to learn, you will never be more than an entry-level dietitian with 30 years' experience! I hope you will continue to read, study, watch, listen, and learn.

Dietitians seem to love to talk about our poor image and what can be done to improve it. Most often, these discussions end with criticism of the ADA for its failure to solve the problem. Many people find it more comfortable to criticize and complain than to contribute. It has always been so. The report of the 1984 Study Commission on Dietetics spoke to this concern and concluded,

> the image of the dietitian will ultimately be determined by the ability of the individual practitioner to present himself/herself as a competent practitioner with a solid academic background, a person who is able to think and reason and participate in decision-making, and a person visibly concerned and involved in the promotion of nutritional well-being for all.

I hope you will want to be that kind of professional.

FACING THE TWENTY-FIRST CENTURY

Today, dietetics is an honored profession with members striving to achieve the highest professional standards of integrity, service, competence, and vision. Two leaders of the profession wrote recently:

> Our profession today is marked by achievement and change. . . . [We] have come a long way in a relatively short period of time. We have become valued professional members of health-care teams and recognized experts in food and nutrition, food service management, and wellness. . . . We need the courage to perceive ourselves succeeding in new roles, to attract a diversity of people to dietetics, and to polish and practice marketing, management, leadership, and sales skills.[33]

Change is rapid in all areas of the dietetics profession—education, research, and practice. The leading issue facing the profession at the present time is healthcare reform. Debate continues over the fundamental changes proposed for the way the nation reimburses healthcare services. Healthcare reform presents both an opportunity and a challenge to the profession.

Increased emphasis is being placed on nutrition and women's health with the recognition of the link between nutrition and the three major diseases that affect women—heart disease, breast cancer, and osteoporosis. The inadequacy of nutrition education in medical schools is another concern—eight of the ten leading diseases in the United States are linked to nutrition. In the commercial/retail foodservice market, dietetic professionals are an underutilized resource.[34] The development of leadership among the members of the profession is another current priority. A number of dynamic and dedicated individuals have emerged to assume leadership roles and will continue to do so as the profession matures.[35]

The gap between consumer nutrition knowledge and behavior presents another opportunity for dietetic practitioners and is the focus of the profession's current market-focused philosophy that individual members serve the profession best by serving the public first.[36] ADA's 1997 Nutrition Trends Survey painted a picture of American consumers—at times exhausted by the barrage of conflicting nutrition information, frustrated by the perceived amount of time required to eat healthfully, feeling that they are doing all they can do regarding nutrition and health, and not as convinced of the importance of diet and nutrition.[37] These findings offer a challenge and an opportunity to members of the profession to "Partner with the Public" to correct misconceptions and offer actionable and credible messages that enable consumers to minimize barriers to eating well and decrease their confusion about nutrition issues.[38]

SUMMARY

Although there is a long history of the relationship of food to health, the profession of dietetics is very young. Much of the progress has been made in the last 100 years. Advances in scientific research, legislation, social and economic factors, military conflicts, and the leadership of some dynamic and dedicated dietitians have contributed to the advancement of the profession.

"Remember the 'old girls,' as they made it possible for us to work for our dream." This statement was made by Marion Mason, Ph.D., R.D., Ruby Winslow Linn Professor of Nutrition, Emerita, at Simmons College in Boston, in an address to the Massachusetts Dietetic Association.[39] It was Lulu Graves, the first president of the ADA, who first sounded the call for teamwork—between physicians and dietitians. "The future of dietetics is assured. It is the privilege of those of us who are now in the work to conduct it along such lines that, in the not very distant future, it will be recognized as part of the medical team."[40]

The increasing diversity of the profession through the years has created the need to broaden the focus of this goal. ADA was founded at a time when most dietitians worked in hospitals. Less than 50 percent of the membership are now employed in this setting.[41] At the dawn of the 21st century, Lulu Graves's quote could be modified to read, It is the privilege of those of us who are now in the work to conduct it along such lines that, in the not very distant future, it will be recognized as the best source for nutrition information and the professionals as those best trained to help consumers make individualized food choices. This comprehensive goal is exemplified in the words inscribed on the ADA seal, adopted in 1940, *Quam Plurimus Prodesse* . . . to benefit as many as possible.

SUGGESTED ACTIVITIES

1. Read one of the autobiographies in *Legends and Legacies* (C. E. Vickery and N. Cotugna, Kendall/Hunt Publishing, 1990) and give an oral report to your class.

2. Secure a very old book on health or cooking from a library or used bookstore. Compare its content to present-day beliefs and practices.

3. Interview a 50-year member of the profession to obtain a personal history of changes that have occurred.

4. Read a journal article chronicling the history of dietetic practice during World War I or II. Two examples are:

    Hodges PAM. Perspective on history: Military dietetics in Europe during World War I. *Journal of American Dietetics Association,* 1993;93:897–900.

Hodges PAM. Perspectives on history: Military dietetics in the Philippines during World War II. *Journal of American Dietetics Association,* 1992;92:840–843.

NOTES

1. Jastrow M. *The Civilization of Babylonia and Assyria.* Philadelphia: J.B. Lippincott Company, 1915.

2. *The Bible* (revised standard version). New York: Collins, 1971.

3. Gove PB, ed. *Webster's Third New International Dictionary.* Springfield, MA: G & C Merriam Co., 1971.

4. Barber MI, ed. *History of the American Dietetic Association* (1917–1959). Philadelphia: J.B. Lippincott Co., 1959.

5. Vehling JD, trans. *Apicius: Cooking and Dining in Imperial Rome.* Chicago: Walter M. Hill, 1936.

6. Whang J. Chinese traditional food therapy. *Journal of the American Dietetic Association,* 1981;78:55–57.

7. Durant W. *Our Oriental Heritage.* New York: Simon & Schuster, 1935.

8. Garrison FH. *An Introduction to the History of Medicine.* 4th ed. Philadelphia: W.B. Saunders Co., 1967.

9. Isch C. A history of hospital fare. In: Beeuwkes AM, Todhunter EN, Weigley ES, eds. *Essays on the History of Nutrition and Dietetics.* Chicago: American Dietetic Association, 1967.

10. De Honesta Voluptate. In: Whitcomb M, ed. *Literary Source Book of the Italian Renaissance.* Philadelphia, 1900.

11. Needham J. Clerks and craftsmen in China and the West. In: *Lectures and Addresses on the History of Science and Technology.* Cambridge, MA: Cambridge University Press, 1970.

12. Rabenn WB. Hospital diets in eighteenth century England. In: Beeuwkes AM, Todhunter EN, Weigley ES, eds. *Essays on the History of Nutrition and Dietetics.* Chicago: American Dietetic Association, 1967.

13. Isch. A history of hospital fare.

14. The American Dietetic Association Study Commission on Dietetics. *A New Look at the Profession of Dietetics.* Chicago: American Dietetic Association, 1984.

15. Cooper LF. Florence Nightingale's contribution to dietetics. In: Beeuwkes AM, Todhunter EN, Weigley ES, eds. *Essays on the History of Nutrition and Dietetics.* Chicago: American Dietetic Association, 1967.

16. Cooper LF. The dietitian and her profession. *Journal of the American Dietetic Association*, 1938;14:751–758.

17. Rorer ST. Early dietetics. *Journal of the American Dietetic Association*, 1934;x:289.

18. Rorer ST. Feeding the sick. *Household News*, 1893;1:69. Rorer ST. How to design a kitchen. *Household News*, 1894;2:17. Rorer ST. Answers to inquiries. *Household News*, 1893;1:13.

19. Weigley ES. Sarah Tyson Rorer: First American dietitian? *Journal of the American Dietetic Association*, 1980;77:11–15.

20. Atwater WO, Bryant AP. *The Chemical Composition of American Food Materials*. U.S. Department of Agriculture Bulletin No. 28. Washington, D.C.: U.S. Government Printing Office, 1896.

21. Corbett FR. The training of dietitians for hospitals. *Journal of Home Economics*, 1909;1:62.

22. Gilson HE. Some historical notes on the development of diet therapy. In Beeuwkes AM, Todhunter EN, Weigley ES, eds. *Essays on the History of Nutrition and Dietetics*. Chicago: American Dietetic Association, 1967.

23. Funk C. The etiology of the deficiency diseases. *Journal of State Medicine*, 1912;341–368.

24. Egan MC. Public health nutrition services: Issues today and tomorrow. *Journal of the American Dietetic Association*, 1980;77:423.

25. Burnett J. *Plenty and Want: A Social History of Diet in England from 1815 to the Present Day*. London: Nelson, 1966.

26. Egan. Public health nutrition services.

27. Egan. Public health nutrition services. Also, Eliot MM, Heseltine, MM. Nutrition in maternal and child health programs. *Nutrition Review*, 1947;533–535.

28. Barber. *History of the American Dietetic Association*.

29. Bray GA. Nutrition in the Humphrey tradition. *Journal of the American Dietetic Association*, 1979;75:116–121.

30. Cross AT. USDA's strategies for the 80s: Nutrition education. *Journal of the American Dietetic Association*, 1980;76:333–337.

31. Ibid.

32. ADA testifies in favor of improving USDA domestic feeding programs. *ADA Courier*, 1993;32:2.

33. Calvert-Finn S, Rinke W. Probing the envelope of Dietetics by transforming challenges into opportunities. *Journal of the American Dietetic Association*, 1989;89:1441–1443.

34. Calvert-Finn S, Bajus B. President's page: 1992–1993 annual report. *Journal of the American Dietetic Association*, 1993;93:1448–1451.

35. Vickery CE, Cotugna N. *Legends and Legacies*. Dubuque, Ia.: Kendall/Hunt Publishing Co., 1990.

36. Coulston A. Ann Coulston, MS, RD, FADA, President, 1998–1999, The American Dietetic Association. *Journal of the American Dietetic Association*, 1998;98:694–695.

37. *1997 Nutrition Trends Survey*. Chicago, Ill: American Dietetic Association; 1997.

38. Coulston A. President's Page: Creating the Future—Partnering with the Public. *Journal of the American Dietetic Association*, 1998;98:817.

39. Fitz PA. President's Page: About 80 years ago. . . . *Journal of the American Dietetic Association*, 1997;97:1160–1161.

40. Cassell JA. *Carry the Flame: The History of The American Dietetic Association*. Chicago, Ill.: American Dietetic Association, 1990.

41. Bryk JA, Soto TK. Report on the 1995 membership database of The American Dietetic Association. *Journal of the American Dietetic Association*, 1997;97:197–203.

PART TWO

The Present

CHAPTER 2

$\diamond$

The Dietetics Profession

WHAT IS DIETETICS?

This is an exciting time to be a nutrition professional. The knowledge that lifestyle choices, such as diet and exercise, can make a dramatic difference in quality of life is becoming more widespread. People are eager for information that can give them an edge in competitive sports, improve physical appearance, make them feel better, and help them live longer, more productive lives. The knowledge that what we eat can dramatically affect our health will create a demand for those who can provide this information. It is predicted that one fifth of all job growth through the year 2005 will occur in healthcare. A number of factors account for this predicted growth. The American population is aging. The Bureau of Labor Statistics predicts that by 2005 the number of Americans over 70 years of age will increase by 11 percent. This "graying of America" will create the need for more specialized medical care, home healthcare, and geriatric specialists. The increasing focus on wellness and preventative medicine by health maintenance organizations (HMOs) and by the public at large has also contributed to the expansion of the healthcare field.[1]

There may be some clouds on the otherwise rosy horizon of the healthcare industry. Cost-containment measures, such as budget cutting, downsizing, realignments, and mergers may affect growth. Many predict that Medicare programs will be reduced, forcing Medicare patients to pay for some home-care costs themselves.[2] However, government surveys of job prospects indicate that healthcare reform will not shrink the workforce.[3]

The three fastest growing career fields are healthcare, computers, and education. Dietetic practitioners are widely employed in each of these fields. Jobs that require a bachelor's degree or higher will grow at a rate almost double that of jobs that require only a high school diploma. By the year 2005, it is predicted that over one fifth of the total workforce will be composed of technicians. A technician is defined as a highly specialized worker who works with physicians, scientists, engineers, and other professionals, as well as with clients, patients, and customers. The technician is further defined as a type of middleperson, between the scientist in the laboratory and the worker on the floor, between the physician and the patient, between the engineer and the factory worker. The technician's realm is where the scientific meets the practical application.[4] In this sense, most dietetic practitioners could be considered technicians.

Perhaps no other profession offers such diversity of opportunity as the field of dietetics does today. Early dietetic practitioners were usually found in an institutional kitchen. Today dietitians can be found almost anywhere. Dietetic practitioners may work in private practice or in a hospital, with patients referred by physicians for help in implementing necessary nutritional modifications. Dietetic practitioners serve as consultants in corporate wellness programs, weight-loss programs, and eating disorder clinics. Professional athletes and athletic teams often have full-time dietitians on their training staffs (Figure 2.1).

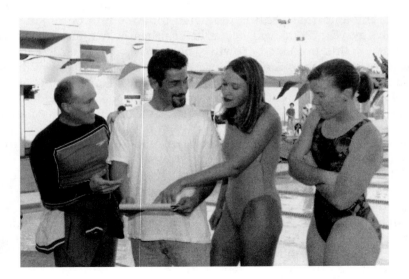

Figure 2.1
A dietitian consults with a coach.

Source: California Dietetic Association. Reprinted with permission.

Dietetic practitioners are also involved in scientific research and education (Figures 2.2 and 2.3). Increasing numbers of dietitians have careers in sales, marketing, and public relations for the food industry, pharmaceutical and computer companies, and equipment manufacturers. They are involved in many areas of community work, especially with pregnant women, women with infants and young children, and the elderly.

Dietetic practitioners are particularly qualified to manage foodservice operations in hospitals, nursing homes, colleges and universities, public schools, commercial restaurants, correctional facilities, catering operations, airline commissaries, and community programs (Figure 2.4).

Although dietetic practitioners are regarded as experts in nutrition, there is still a lack of recognition from the public. And while the American public has increased its knowledge and understanding of foods and nutrition, misinformation still abounds. Popular magazines are full of attention-grabbing, but inaccurate, advice. Health-food stores promote the sale of supposed "super nutrients" to the tune of billions of dollars a year. The general public lacks the educational background

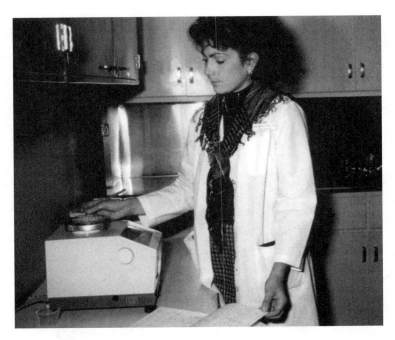

Figure 2.2
A dietitian conducting food science research.

Source: VA Greater Los Angeles Healthcare System at the West L.A. Healthcare Center, Food and Nutrition. Reprinted with permission.

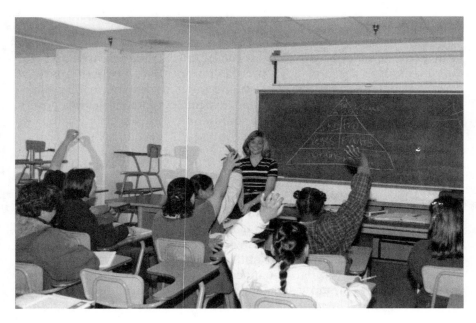

Figure 2.3
A dietitian teaches the Food Guide Pyramid to a class of young children.

Source: California Dietetic Association. Reprinted with permission.

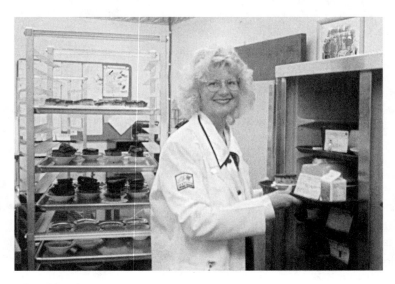

Figure 2.4
A dietary manager checks patient trays for accuracy.

Source: Photo courtesy of Doris Douglas, C.D.M.

to discern a good study from a poor one. Many people still don't know that you can't believe everything you read.

The basis of dietetics is the firm belief that optimal nutrition is essential for the health and well-being of every person. This is why dietetics is an integral component of the healthcare field. Nutritional support helps return patients to health and keep them that way. A team effort by doctors, nurses, and dietitians is usually necessary to return a patient to health.

The words *food* and *nutrition* are not synonymous. Food is the main source of nourishment, which is influenced by a complex array of internal and external factors. When food cannot be used to achieve nutrition, intravenous feeding or total parenteral nutrition (TPN) become important.

Societal needs are best served by having a population that is adequately nourished. Dietetics serves people by offering correct and current information so that individuals can make their own choices. The education, training, and knowledge of dietitians make them uniquely qualified to help individuals and society to meet nutritional needs.

WHAT IS A PROFESSION?

What is a profession, and how does dietetics qualify as a profession? One generic definition might be "A profession is an occupation for which preliminary training is intellectual in character, involving knowledge and learning as distinguished from mere skill, which is pursued largely for others and not merely for one's self, and in which financial return is not an accepted measure of success." The goals committee of The American Dietetic Association (ADA) interprets a profession as a calling requiring

- Specialized knowledge and often long and intensive preparation
- Instruction in skills and methods as well as scientific, historical, or scholarly principles underlying such skills and methods
- Maintenance, by force of organization or concerted opinion, of high standards of achievement and conduct
- Commitment of its members to continued study
- A kind of work that has as its primary purpose the rendering of a public service.

A professional is one who represents or belongs to a profession.[5]

HOW IS DIETETICS A PROFESSION?

Five main characteristics of dietetic practice qualify it for professional status:

1. A specialized body of knowledge
2. Specialized services rendered to society
3. An obligation for service to the client that overrides personal considerations
4. Concern for competence and honor among the practitioners
5. An obligation for continuing education, research, and sharing of knowledge for the common good

A dietitian has been defined as "a professional person who is a translator of the science and art of foods, nutrition, and dietetics in the service of people—whether individually or in families or larger groups; healthy or sick; and at all stages of the life cycle."[6] Dietetic practice is defined as the application of principles derived from the integration of knowledge of food, nutrition, biochemistry, physiology, management, and behavioral and social science to achieve and maintain the health of people.[7] See Figure 2.5 for a graphic depiction of the different fields integrated by dietitians.[8]

SPECIALTY AREAS AND NEW EMPLOYMENT OPPORTUNITIES

Here is a listing of some of the employment opportunities related to nutrition and foods:

Clinical dietitian (including specialty areas such as renal, pediatric, nutrition support, etc.)

Commercial foodservice administrator

Community college educator

Consulting nutritionist

Consumer and public relations specialist for food company

Diet counselor

Educational representative for business

Extension service 4-H coordinator

Extension service home advisor

Food advertising consultant

Food analyst/technologist

Food broker

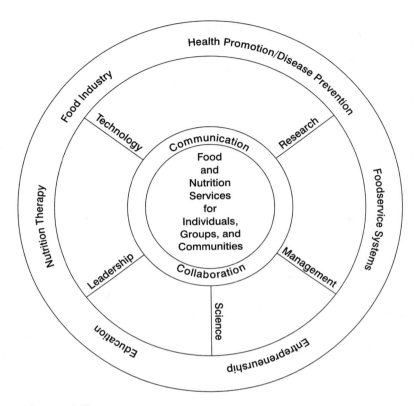

Figure 2.5
Model for dietetics practice.

Source: Gilmore CJ, O'Sullivan Maillet J, Mitchell BE. Determining Educational Preparation Based on Job Competencies of Entry-Level Dietetics Practitioners. Copyright The American Dietetic Association. Reprinted by permission from JOURNAL OF THE AMERICAN DIETETIC ASSOCIATION, Vol. 97(3):306–316, 1997.

Food editor

Food journalist

Food photography specialist

Food quality assurance specialist

Food research and marketing specialist

Food scientist

Food science educator

Foodservice administrator for airline or cruise line

Food stylist

Home economist for food or equipment business

Home healthcare dietitian

Hospital foodservice administrator

Marketing specialist for food or nutrition company

Nutrition educator

Nutrition researcher

Peace Corps representative

Private practitioner

Product development researcher

Public health nutritionist

Rehabilitation consultant

Research chemist

Restaurant foodservice administrator

Sales representative for food or equipment

School foodservice administrator

Sports nutritionist

Taste panel coordinator

Test kitchen scientist[9]

This list is by no means exhaustive, but it shows the breadth of opportunities that are available to someone who has training in foods and nutrition. The educational requirements for these positions varies from some college work to an advanced degree. Many do not require any credential.

Because of the increasingly specialized nature of dietetic practice, the leadership of the ADA developed Dietetic Practice Groups (DPGs).[10] DPGs provide a way for members of the ADA to network within their area or areas of interest and practice. Currently, there are 29 DPGs. These are described in Chapter 7 (pp. 138–142).

The ADA is the oldest and most prominent professional organization for dietitians, and it is discussed at length in Chapter 7. Among the most important functions of the ADA is the development of Standards of Professional Practice, outlining a dietetic practitioner's responsibilities for providing quality nutritional care. The standards provide individual practitioners with a systematic plan for implementing, evaluating, and adjusting performance in any area of practice. See Chapter 6 for a discussion of the standards and for the text of the standards (see Figure 6.11).[11] Chapter 6 also discusses ethics and the profession of dietetics (pp. 110–118).

Another important function of the ADA is its recognition of excellence in practice through the awards given annually by the ADA and by

PROFILE

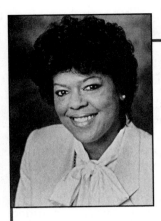

Bettye Nowlin, M.S., R.D.

POSITION
  Manager, Public Affairs, Dairy Council of California
EDUCATION
  B.S. Tennessee Agricultural and Industrial University, Nashville
  M.P.H. University of California at Los Angeles
ROUTE TO REGISTRATION
  Dietetic internship

◆ **Professional Involvement**
One of sixteen original Ambassadors for the ADA
Director-at-Large, Board of Directors, the ADA
Member, Nominating Committee, the ADA
Numerous state and local dietetic association offices and committees

◆ **Honors and Awards Received**
Medallion Award, the ADA
ADA Foundation's Award for Excellence in Practice for Community Nutrition
California Dietetic Association's Distinguished Service Award

◆ **Words of Wisdom for Future Dietetics Professionals**
During my career, I have held all kinds of positions, including clinical dietitian at Cook County Hospital, administrative dietitian at Michael Reese Hospital and Medical Center, high school home economics teacher, and public health nutritionist, all in Chicago. I then moved to Los Angeles, where I became involved as a nutrition consultant with Head Start and the Senior Feeding Program. I also worked as nutrition education consultant, program director, and now manager of public affairs for the Dairy Council of California. The diversity that is available in this profession is incredible!

Being involved in my profession has always been a priority. This involvement has contributed much to my personal and professional development. I encourage students to become involved in the student dietetic association at their university and to volunteer for activities within their local dietetic association. Attending local, state, and national dietetics meetings are a wonderful way to network and learn more about the profession. Volunteering for roles is mutually beneficial, as it helps build leadership skills and confidence.

Choosing dietetics as a career has allowed me to do the things that give me pleasure and satisfaction and to work and interact with colleagues that I care about. It doesn't get any better than that!

affiliated state associations of ADA. See Chapter 7 for a list and description of these awards (pp. 143–146).

ROLE DELINEATION STUDIES

To identify the major and specific responsibilities that dietetic practitioners must assume to ensure quality care, the ADA periodically conducts empirical practice analyses. Three role delineation studies, conducted in 1983 and 1984, focused on what practitioners in clinical dietetics, community dietetics, and foodservice systems management were doing and what they ought to be doing.[12] A 1989 study measured what practitioners in a variety of settings actually do, at entry-level and beyond. No measures of quality, correctness, or efficacy were included in the 1989 study.[13] A practice audit conducted in 1995 was designed to update the earlier study, to provide more extensive analyses of the differences in levels of responsibility in different areas of dietetics practice, and to determine which aspects of practice are likely to change in the next few years.[14] The results of the study are not being used just to define appropriate responsibilities and knowledge bases for competent dietetic practice. The educational component of the profession will use the data collected to update knowledge and performance requirements and develop curriculum. The practice component of the profession will use the study to revise practice standards and develop outcome criteria for quality assurance. And the certification component of the profession will use the study as a basis for test specifications for the registration examinations.[15]

SUMMARY

"The world is happier, healthier, [and] better off because of the work you do," proclaimed Rabbi Harold S. Kushner to the dietetic professionals gathered at an ADA Annual Meeting.[16] The work of dietetics is considered a profession because it requires a specialized body of knowledge; because members render specialized services to society; because their obligations to serve override personal considerations; and because members consider competence, honor, continuing education, research, and sharing of knowledge for the common good to be necessary.

Dietetic practice encompasses nutrition therapy, the food industry, health promotion/disease prevention, foodservice systems, entrepreneurship, and education. Drawing on their training and knowledge in the fields of science, leadership, technology, research, and management, dietetic professionals communicate and collaborate to provide food and nutrition services for individuals, groups, and communities.

The ADA has developed DPGs to allow members to network and increase their knowledge within their particular area of practice (see Chapter 7); annual awards for excellence in specific areas of practice (see Chapter 7); and standards of practice that outline a dietetic practitioner's responsibilities for providing quality nutritional care (see Chapter 6).

SUGGESTED ACTIVITIES

1. Choose one of the DPGs you might be interested in joining later in your career. If possible, attend one of the meetings of this practice group at an annual meeting of ADA or at a regional meeting. Or, interview a member of the practice group to find out what the practice group does to benefit the profession and individual members.

2. Add to the list of specialty areas of dietetic practice included in the chapter by either listing positions you know exist or by developing areas of practice or positions you would be interested in personally. Be creative!

3. Visit the ADA Web site at www.eatright.org to verify the accuracy of information in this chapter. Has anything changed since the chapter was written?

NOTES

1. *The Top 100: The Fastest Growing Careers for the 21st Century.* Chicago, Ill.: Ferguson Publishing Co., 1998.

2. Ibid.

3. Bureau of Labor Statistics. Health-care reforms won't shrink the workforce. *Business and Health,* May 1995;19.

4. *The Top 100.*

5. The American Dietetic Association Committee on Goals of Education for Dietetics. Goals of the lifetime education of the dietitian. *Journal of the American Dietetic Association,* 1969;54:91–93.

6. Galbraith A. Excellence defined. *Journal of the American Dietetic Association,* 1975;67:211.

7. South ML. Charting for the changing scene. In: Vaden AG, ed. *Charting for the Changing Scene.* Chicago, Ill.: American Dietetic Association, 1981.

8. Gilmore CJ, O'Sullivan Maillet J, Mitchell BE. Determining educational preparation based on job competencies of entry-level

dietetics practitioners. *Journal of The American Dietetic Association,* 1997:97:306–316.

9. American Dietetic Association. *Set Your Sights: Your Future in Dietetics.* Chicago, Ill.: The American Dietetic Association, 1991.

10. American Dietetic Association. *Dietetic Practice Groups.* Chicago, Ill.: The American Dietetic Association, 1998.

11. American Dietetic Association. The American Dietetic Association Standards of Professional Practice for Dietetics Professionals. *Journal of the American Dietetic Association,* 1998;98:83–87.

12. American Dietetic Association. *Role Delineation and Verification for Entry-Level Positions in Community Dietetics.* Chicago: The American Dietetic Association, 1983; American Dietetic Association. *Role Delineation and Verification for Entry-Level Positions in Food Service Systems Management.* Chicago: The American Dietetic Association, 1983; American Dietetic Association. *Role Delineation and Verification for Entry-Level Positions in Clinical Dietetics.* Chicago, Ill.: The American Dietetic Association, 1984.

13. American Dietetic Association. *Role Delineation for Registered Dietitians and Entry-Level Dietetic Technicians.* Chicago, Ill.: The American Dietetic Association, 1990.

14. Kane MT, Cohen AS, Smith ER, Lewis C, Reidy C. 1995 Commission on Dietetic Registration Dietetics Practice Audit. *Journal of the American Dietetic Association,* 1996;96:1292–1301.

15. ADA. *Role Delineation.*

16. ADA. *Set Your Sights.*

CHAPTER 3

◆

Joining Together: The Team Approach

In all health care settings more work is being done by versatile and flexible multidisciplinary teams that plan, implement, and review cases (Figure 3.1). Members are valued for their ability to help the team with a "flexible eye" in making judgments and pitching in to do what needs to be done. The most valued members are those with a global view of health and proficiency in a greater number of competencies. Teams reduce costs by using fewer employees, using them synergistically, and pushing care toward lower-paid practitioners.[1]

The need to be multiskilled and cross trained is increasing.

Long gone are the days of the family doctor acting alone to treat disease. A career in healthcare is no longer limited to being either a doctor or nurse. The healthcare system in the United States is one of the most sophisticated and complex in the world. The increase in number of elderly people (there are now three million more people over the age of 75 than there were five years ago); rampant shortages in the healthcare workforce; specialized treatments requiring complex technology; increasing emphasis on preventive healthcare; and an increased understanding of the cost benefits of a healthy workforce all create very positive prospects for anyone entering a healthcare career.

Healthcare services are expected to increase by 30 percent and account for 3.1 million new jobs from 1996 to 2006, the largest numerical increase of any industry. In an attempt to contain costs, the healthcare industry will increasingly shift patients out of hospitals and into outpatient facilities, nursing homes, and home healthcare.[2]

The explosion of knowledge in science has led to a corresponding explosion in the number of healthcare professions that demand specialized knowledge and skills. The term *allied health* is used to describe a cluster of roles in the healthcare system that assist, facili-

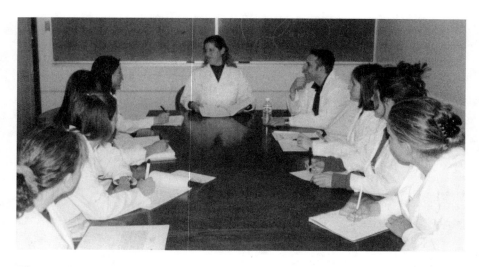

Figure 3.1
An informal medical team meeting.

Source: Courtesy of Pepperdine University, Malibu, California.

tate, and complement the work of physicians and other healthcare specialists. The American Society of Allied Health Professions lists more than 85 different health service careers.[3] For example, the data acquired by laboratory technicians plays a crucial role in the detection, diagnosis, and treatment of disease. The medical records administrator collects, analyzes, and manages information that steers the healthcare industry. The rehabilitation process for a patient often requires the combined efforts of physical therapists, a medical social worker, occupational therapists, and dietitians. The hospital pharmacist works with nurses, doctors, and dietitians to provide quality patient care. These specialty areas free highly skilled medical practitioners to perform the tasks they alone are qualified to do.

Along with the expansion in number of allied health professions, there has been an expansion in the number of work settings. Fitness centers, gyms, and spas are examples of nontraditional settings where dietitians are finding employment today.

The high demand, combined with stability, excellent starting salaries, mobility, and flexibility make a health services career very attractive to those with the desire to help others. The attributes and skills that are considered characteristic of successful healthcare professionals are enjoyment of the basic biological sciences; intellectual capacity to solve problems; flexibility; patience; investigative skills;

respect for others as human beings; effective communication skills; counseling skills; diagnostic and teaching skills; research design skills; computer skills; an understanding of technical equipment; and the ability to be a team player.

The concept of the team approach in the healthcare setting, encompassing a number of health professionals, has been increasingly encouraged in the past 30 years in order to provide patients/clients with safe, timely, and effective care.

THE HISTORY OF THE HEALTHCARE TEAM CONCEPT

The concept of the healthcare team emerged after World War II with an increased social awareness and expectations of healthcare for all. Disabled veterans returning from the war needed more than traditional medical treatment for their physical disabilities: They needed all kinds of help to return to the community as socially and economically useful citizens. The trend toward sharing responsibilities that had formerly been the sole purview of the physician and/or nurse has had a major impact on quality of care, healthcare costs, and the organization and delivery of healthcare.[4]

TEAMWORK

Teamwork is the close, cooperative effort of several people to use their special skills and knowledge to meet the needs of the client/patient more efficiently, completely, competently, and considerately than would be possible by individual, independent action.[5] An important, but often forgotten, member of the team is the client/patient. Educating and including the client/patient in the team communication process is critically important.[6] Because the ultimate responsibility for client/patient care rests with the physician, it is the physician who assumes leadership of most healthcare teams. Other members of the team vary depending on the needs of the client/patient.

To function effectively, healthcare teams must be able to differentiate between those roles that are unique to each discipline and those that are shared. Team members function independently when they have unique competencies, knowledge, and experiences. Delegated functioning occurs when the team has varying levels and types of training. Collaborative functioning is used when an overlap in competencies allows for a common base for judgment and decision making.[7]

A clinical dietitian doing a patient discharge diet instruction is functioning independently. A delegated function for this same dietitian would be the implementation of a physician-prescribed diet order. An example of a collaborative, multidisciplinary approach would be the implementation of a weight-control program involving a physician, dietitian, exercise physiologist, laboratory technician, and psychologist.[8] Diseases that have systemic effects are natural candidates for the collaborative, multidisciplinary team approach. For example, care for diabetic patients often involves a primary care physician, endocrinologist, dietitian, nurse/nurse practitioner, ophthalmologist, podiatrist, health educator, and others.

Teamwork may be problematic if roles are not clearly defined, communication is not adequate and open, members fail to be good team players, and team goals are not clearly defined. Accurate and timely sharing of data is a key element in the effectiveness of the team effort. Team conferences, where all team members share information and participate in decision making, are the preferred approach.

MEMBERS OF THE HEALTHCARE TEAM

There are more than 85 possible members of the healthcare team! A few are highlighted in the following section. Members of the dietetic team form a subset of the larger healthcare team and are discussed first. Members of the dietetic team can most often be found working in the institutional healthcare setting. Dietitians, dietetic technicians, and dietary managers are the primary positions that make up the dietetic team. In recent years, healthcare issues such as labor shortages, cost containment, and quality assurance have forced the dietetic team to be better coordinated and to delegate less specialized, more routine tasks to less highly trained personnel.

Members of the dietetic team receive formal training in nutrition and foods. The demand for personnel with this background is greater than the supply. The number of employment opportunities continues to expand. A wide variety of settings for such work exists, and the responsibilities encompassed by each job are as varied as the settings.

The Dietitians

Dietitians are highly qualified professionals who are recognized experts on food and nutrition. The educational requirements to become a dietitian are described in Chapter 4. The American Dietetic Association (ADA) is the primary professional association for dietitians and dietetic technicians. Dietitians work in a wide variety of settings, most of which fall into seven major categories, discussed next.

Business Dietitians Business dietitians work in areas such as food manufacturing, advertising, and marketing. Dietitians who work for food manufacturers or grocery chains may analyze the nutrition content of foods for labeling purposes or marketing efforts. They may also prepare literature for distribution to customers and write articles for the news media. To satisfy consumers' growing interest in nutrition, dietitians are employed by businesses to develop new products, sell and market products, and develop public relations and advertising programs. Many entrepreneurial dietitians have developed a product, product line, or a service themselves, and built a company to market and sell the products or services.

Clinical Dietitians Clinical dietitians provide nutritional services for patients in hospitals, nursing homes, clinics, health maintenance organizations (HMOs), doctors' offices, and other healthcare facilities. They assess patients' nutritional needs, develop and implement nutrition programs, and evaluate and report the results. They are a vital part of the healthcare team, working with doctors and other healthcare professionals to coordinate nutritional intake with other treatment such as medications.

Many clinical dietitians specialize in one area of practice. Diabetes, heart disease, pediatrics, gerontology, kidney disease, the critically ill, and obesity are some of the areas in which clinical dietitians specialize. Nutritional care of the critically ill, for example, involves overseeing the preparation of custom-mixed, high-nutrition formulas for patients requiring tube or intravenous feedings. Clinical dietitians working with diabetics teach patients how to establish and adhere to a long-term nutrition program and how to monitor blood glucose levels.

In addition to assessing nutrition needs and developing treatment plans, clinical dietitians have administrative and managerial duties. The clinical dietitian in a small nursing home or hospital may run the foodservice department. In larger facilities, clinical dietitians may supervise dietetic technicians and other support staff such as patient service supervisors, diet clerks, and clerical personnel.

Community Dietitians Community dietitians reach out to the public to teach, monitor, and advise individuals and groups in their efforts to prevent disease and promote good health. They are employed by international organizations; federal, state and local governments; food businesses; and trade associations. A variety of public, private, and volunteer organizations concerned with international health employ community nutritionists. The United Nations and the Peace Corps are just two such organizations. The U.S. Department of Agriculture, U.S. Department of Health and Human Services, and the public health division of state and local governments employ community nutritionists to plan and carry out programs to address nutritional problems of targeted groups. The WIC program is one example. The main responsibility of community nutritionists employed by food businesses and associations is nutrition education. For example, the dairy industry has organized large-scale nutrition education programs for schoolchildren and other groups (see Figures 3.2 and 3.3).

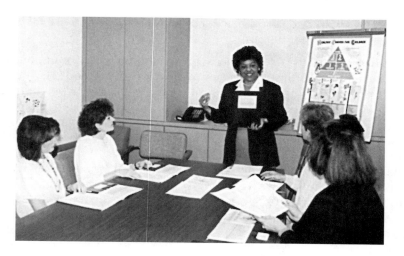

Figure 3.2
A dairy council dietitian conducts a nutrition education
program.

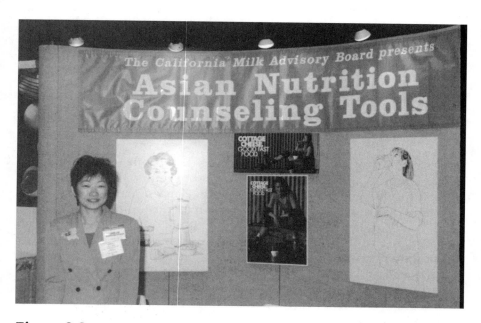

Figure 3.3
A community dietitian displays counseling tools at a
professional meeting.

Source: California Dietetic Association. Reprinted with permission.

Community dietitians evaluate individual needs, establish nutritional care plans, and communicate the principles of good nutrition in a way individuals and their families can understand. Teaching is a very large component of the community dietitian's job. Topics run the gamut from grocery shopping to the preparation of infant formula, from menu planning for diabetics to alcoholism, from breast-feeding to hypertension.

Consultant Dietitians   Consultant dietitians may be self-employed in their own private practice or under contract to one or more healthcare facilities. In private practice, the consultant dietitian performs nutrition screening and assessment of clients, who are often referred by a physician. Weight loss is the most common diet-related concern of clients who seek a private practice dietitian. Consultant dietitians under contract to healthcare facilities provide expert advice on foodservice management issues such as menu planning, budgeting, cost control, portion control, sanitation, and safety, and they also monitor clinical nutritional care (Figure 3.4).

Educator Dietitians   Educator dietitians teach future dietitians, dietetic technicians, dietary managers, doctors, nurses, dentists, chefs, and others the science of foods and nutrition. They are employed by uni-

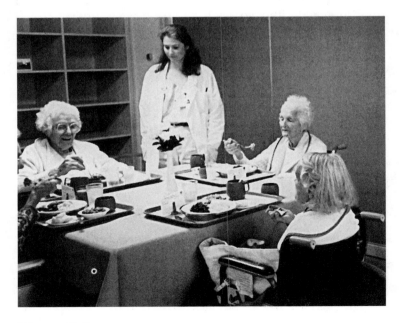

Figure 3.4
A consultant dietitian checking a meal service.

versities, four-year colleges, community colleges, technical schools, and dietetic internship programs. Although education is a major component of most dietitians' job responsibilities, this category is for those who are employed by an educational institution or program, rather than an organization whose primary responsibility is healthcare.

Management Dietitians   Management dietitians play a very important role wherever food is served. They are responsible for large-scale meal planning and preparation in such places as hospitals, nursing homes and retirement residences, company cafeterias, correctional facilities, elementary and secondary schools, food factories, colleges and universities, transportation companies, restaurants, the military, and recreational facilities.

The management dietitian supervises the planning, preparation, and service of meals; selects, trains, and directs other dietitians, foodservice supervisors, and foodservice workers; budgets for and purchases food, equipment, and supplies; enforces sanitary and safety regulations; and prepares records and reports (Figure 3.5).

Dietitians who direct food and nutrition departments also decide on departmental policies and coordinate food and nutrition services with the activities of other departments. The use of computer programs to adjust recipes, prepare purchase orders, cost recipes and menus, keep inventory records, prepare financial reports, conduct nutritional analyses, and so on has simplified many of the routine functions of management dietetics.

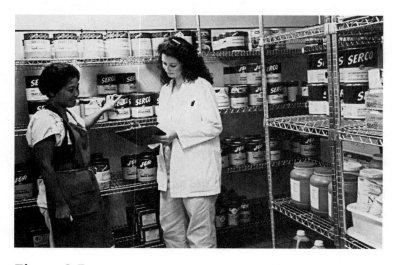

Figure 3.5
A management dietitian at work.

PROFILE

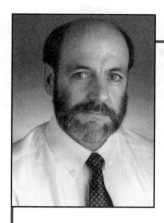

Peter Beyer, M.S., R.D., L.D.

POSITION
> R.D./graduate faculty member, combined intern-
> ship/master's degree program, University of
> Kansas Medical Center, Kansas City, KS

EDUCATION
> B.S. Central Missouri State University,
> Warrensburg, MO
> M.S. University of Missouri Medical Center,
> Columbia, MO

ROUTE TO REGISTRATION
> Dietetic internship

◆ **Professional Involvement**
Chair, Commission on Dietetic Registration
Member of two ADA role delineation committees
Member of two ADA strategic planning committees
Member, Advanced Level Practice Committee
Member, Clinical Indicators Task Force
Member, Ethics Committee
Member, Standards of Practice Implementation Task Force
American Society of Parenteral and Enteral Nutrition
Delegate from Kansas to ADA's House of Delegates
Presented over 250 times to local, state, and national audiences on a
variety of topics

◆ **Honors and Awards Received**
Recognized Young Dietitian of the Year
Distinguished Teaching Award from the University of Kansas Medical
Center, School of Allied Health
Outstanding Dietitian of the Year, Kansas City Dietetic Association
Excellence in Practice Award in Clinical Nutrition from the ADA Foun-
dation
Outstanding Dietetics Educator from ADA's Commission on Accredita-
tion/Approval of Dietetics Education
1998 Recipient of the Outstanding Graduate Award from the Depart-
ment of Human Ecology, Central Missouri State University

◆ **Words of Wisdom for Future Dietetics Professionals**
Thinking back to things that helped me learn to do a better job with
patients and students and helped me in my own development, I realize
that the key was to continually push myself to understand and, subse-

quently, teach others about the fascinating things I've learned in my
profession. I often volunteered to participate in, review, or carry out
projects that either required that I learn a great deal before my participation or that resulted in my growth simply because I was working with
really good people. Each time I became involved with a committee or a
task force, or was asked to present or write, I hoped that I contributed
as much as I learned in the process. I think that I'm finally getting to
that point that I've learned enough, had enough experiences, and have
made enough mistakes that I can see a little more clearly how much
there is to know and what things are important—that is, at least in
some aspects of our diverse profession. It's kinda fun!

Research Dietitians   Research dietitians work for government agencies,
food or pharmaceutical companies, academic medical centers, or educational institutions. Using the scientific method and analytical techniques, they conduct studies that range from pure to applied science.
Often, research is conducted collaboratively with physicians, exercise
physiologists, chemists, food technologists, and researchers from
other disciplines. Research dietitians may explore the way the body
uses a particular food or the interaction of drugs and diet. They may
investigate the nutritional needs of individuals with different diseases
or ways to reduce the risk of disease. Research in the managerial
arena may involve the effectiveness of various foodservice systems or
the efficiency of different types of foodservice equipment.

Dietetic Technicians   Dietetic technicians complete a two-year associate
degree in an ADA-approved dietetic technician program that combines
both classroom and supervised practice experiences. They are then eligible to take the registration examination for dietetic technicians. Individuals who pass the exam may then use the initials *D.T.R.*, for
Dietetic Technician, Registered, after their names.

Dietetic technicians work in a wide variety of settings and assume
an even-wider variety of responsibilities. Dietetic technicians are found
in hospitals, public health nutrition programs, long-term care facilities, child nutrition and school lunch programs, nutrition programs
for the elderly, and foodservice management. Screening patients to
identify nutritional problems, modifying menus, providing patient education and counseling to individuals and groups, developing menus
and recipes, supervising foodservice personnel, purchasing food, con-

ducting inventory, and maintaining computer systems are the most commonly performed functions of a dietetic technician.

Dietary Managers Dietary managers are members of the Dietary Managers Association (DMA). While no legal relationship exists between the ADA and the DMA, a very close working relationship has always been in existence. Educational requirements, job settings and responsibilities, and the DMA are described in detail in Chapter 8.

Other Members of the Healthcare Team

Physicians Required training for physicians includes a four-year postgraduate medical degree (either an M.D. or a D.O.). Medical schools in the United States have specific undergraduate entrance requirements including mathematics, sciences, and humanities. Entrance to medical school is very competitive and based on undergraduate grade-point average; the results of a standardized medical school entrance exam; letters of recommendation; and community service, volunteer, or research experience.

Medical school includes two years of basic medical science followed by two years of clinical training. The clinical training concentrates heavily on the daily care of hospitalized patients. During these two years, medical students begin to explore areas of specialization in medicine. Following graduation from medical school, most doctors complete a residency in a specialty, which lasts three to five years. A fellowship may follow the residency program if a doctor wants to train in a subspecialty area. For example, a residency in pediatrics could be followed by a fellowship in neonatology (care of newborns including premature infants), pediatric cardiology (the heart and circulatory system), pediatric neurology (the brain and nervous system), pediatric hematology (the blood), pediatric oncology (cancer and tumors), pediatric gastroenterology (the digestive system), or pediatric nephrology (the kidneys).

A primary care physician provides the majority of care to well and sick patients. The primary care specialties are pediatrics (infants and children), family practice, geriatrics (the elderly), and obstetrics/gynecology. Other physician specialties are listed here.

Cardiologists Cardiologists diagnose and treat cardiovascular defects and diseases. They are concerned with the structure and function of the heart and blood vessels and with the circulation of blood throughout the body.

Oncologists Oncology is concerned with neoplastic growth (abnormal new growth of cells and tissues), including the cause and the pattern of the abnormality.

Neurologists Neurology is an internal medicine specialty that deals with disorders of the human brain, spinal cord, peripheral nerves, and muscles. Neurologists care for patients with a myriad of disorders such as pain, weakness in the arms or legs, or memory loss.

Pathologists Pathologists provide and interpret laboratory information to help solve diagnostic problems and monitor the effects of therapy for other medical specialists.

Endocrinologists An endocrinologist diagnoses and treats diseases of the hormone-producing glandular system—including the pituitary, thyroid, parathyroid, adrenals, and gonads—and the insulin-producing cells of the pancreas. Endocrinologists also treat patients with metabolic disorders.

Surgeons Surgeons deal with problems by using operative procedures. The problems may be mechanical or structural (e.g., hernias, fractures, or ulcers); biological (e.g., ulcer); or metabolic (e.g., an islet cell tumor of the pancreas, which causes the pancreas to secrete too much insulin). Surgical subspecialties include gastrointestinal (digestive tract), plastic surgery, vascular (blood vessels), cardiothoracic (heart and chest), pediatric (children), endocrine (glands), orthopedic (bones and joints), urology (kidney and bladder), neurologic (brain and nervous system), otolaryngology (ear, nose, and throat), gynecology (female organs), hand, trauma and burn, oncology (cancer), and transplantation (transplanted organs).

Psychiatrists Psychiatrists treat patients with mental illnesses and are able to prescribe medicines for illnesses such as depression and schizophrenia.

Podiatrists Podiatrists specialize in the care and treatment of the human foot.

Ophthalmologists Ophthalmology is the branch of medicine dealing with the structure, function, and diseases of the eye, including medical and surgical treatment of its defects and diseases.

Osteopathic Physicians Osteopathy is a system of medical practice based on a theory that diseases are due chiefly to loss of structural integrity, which can be restored by manipulation of the parts supplemented by therapeutic measures (e.g., medicine, physical therapy, or surgery).

Osteopathic physicians use the title D.O., which stands for doctor of osteopathy.

Chiropractors   A doctor of chiropractic (D.C.) has completed a minimum of two years of college credit toward a baccalaureate degree and three-and-a-half to four years at a chiropractic college. Chiropractic care emphasizes a holistic approach to health and is based on the premise that the relationship between structure and function in the human body (particularly of the spinal column and nervous system) is a significant health factor. Chiropractors believe that when the spinal column is out of alignment, the body's natural defenses to disease and illness are lowered. Chiropractors realign the spinal column so that the body stays in a state of homeostasis, or balance.

Nurses   Nurses are active in the prevention of illness in clinics, industry, and public health; the care of patients in emergency and intensive-care situations; general nursing care in hospitals and long-term care settings; and the care of patients in their own homes. There are more than 100 nursing specialties. The specialty may focus on a specific disease, organ/system, setting, scope of practice, patient age, criticalness of patient condition, or technology.

Nurse Practitioners   Nurse practitioners are registered nurses with advanced formal education. Most have a master's degree in nursing and are certified by a national professional association. Working in collaboration with physicians and other healthcare team members, nurse practitioners obtain medical histories and perform physical exams; diagnose and treat common health problems; diagnose, treat, and monitor chronic diseases; order and interpret lab work and x-rays; prescribe medications and other treatments; provide family planning, prenatal care, well-baby and child care, and health maintenance care; conduct patient and family education and counseling programs; provide referrals to healthcare team members; and, in some states, prescribe medicines.

Pharmacists   Hospital pharmacists monitor a patient's drug therapy, prepare intravenous medications and feedings, oversee drug administration, and make purchasing decisions. Pharmacists are important members of many healthcare teams.

Social Workers   The field of social work is incredibly broad. A bachelor of arts in social work is always required; a master's degree in social work (M.S.W.) is increasingly required. The undergraduate degree is broad-based, with elective courses in substance abuse, grief, and race and gender issues. Graduate programs explore human behavior, mental disorders, and methods of intervention and psychotherapy in greater depth.

Physical Therapists   Physical therapists design and administer rehabilitative exercise programs for people with injuries or disabilities that impact their daily functioning (Figure 3.6).

Athletic Trainers   Athletic trainers provide services such as injury prevention, recognition, immediate care, treatment, and rehabilitation of athletic trauma.

Medical Assistants   Medical assistants assist physicians in their offices or other medical settings by performing a variety of administrative and clinical duties.

Medical Laboratory Technicians/Technologists   Under the supervision of a pathologist, a "lab tech" performs lab tests, using precision instruments, on

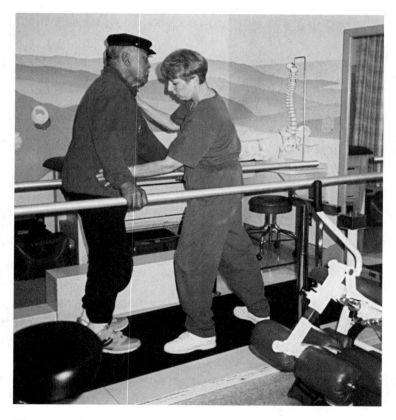

Figure 3.6
A physical therapist assists a stroke patient whose
balance and gait have been impaired.

blood, tissues, and body fluids to detect, diagnose, and treat diseases. Medical lab technologists are able to perform the same duties as a technician and can also perform more complex analyses, discrimination, and correction of errors. Histologic technicians/technologists specialize in the preparation of body tissues for laboratory analysis.

Medical Records Administrators   A medical record comprises the complete and permanent documents maintained for every person treated in a medical facility. Medical records administrators manage the medical record in compliance with medical, administrative, ethical, and legal requirements. The medical records technician (MRT) is responsible for maintaining the medical records.

Nuclear Medicine Technologists   A nuclear medicine technologist assists a nuclear medicine physician. These physicians use the nuclear properties of radioactive and stable nuclides to make diagnostic evaluations of the anatomic or physiologic conditions of the body.

Occupational Therapists   Occupational therapists and their assistants provide service to individuals whose abilities to cope with the tasks of living are threatened or impaired by developmental deficits, the aging process, poverty and cultural differences, physical injury or illness, or psychological and social disability (Figures 3.7 and 3.8). The therapy is directed toward teaching adaptive skills and enhancing performance capacity to achieve optimal function, prevent disability, or maintain health. The goal is the highest possible functional independence for self-care, work, and leisure.

Physician Assistants   The physician assistant (P.A.), under the supervision of a physician, performs diagnostic, therapeutic, preventive, and health maintenance services. Duties include, but are not limited to, the following: performing complete physical examinations; performing and/or interpreting routine diagnostic procedures; giving injections and immunizations; suturing and wound care; and instructing and counseling patients.

Radiologic Technologists   Under the supervision of radiation oncologists, "rad techs" administer radiation therapy to patients. Radiographers, also under the supervision of qualified physicians, provide patient service using imaging modalities.

Respiratory Therapists   The respiratory therapist and respiratory therapy technician evaluate all data to determine the appropriate respiratory care for a patient and conduct the therapeutic procedures to carry out this plan.

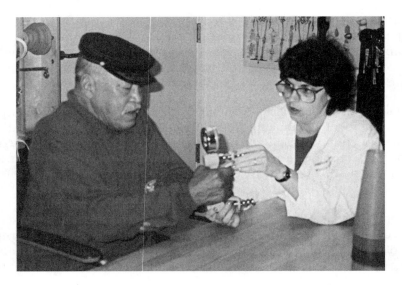

Figure 3.7
An occupational therapist tests a stroke patient's grip.

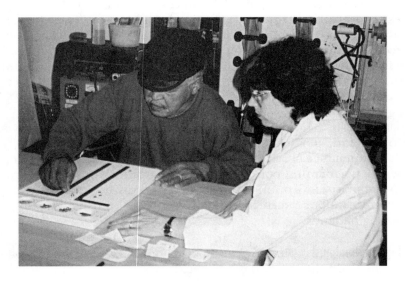

Figure 3.8
Under the watchful eye of an occupational therapist, a stroke patient completes an exercise to improve hand–eye coordination and manual dexterity.

SUMMARY

Teamwork is important in the healthcare professions today, due in part to the enormous number of people employed in these careers. The team approach is an effective way of dealing with the fragmentation of care that may occur due to specialization.

Dietitians, dietetic technicians, and dietary managers are the members of the dietetic team. They have all received formal training in foods and nutrition, and as a team, they work in a wide variety of settings. Dietitians, who are recognized experts in food and nutrition, are found working in the business, clinical, community, consulting, education, management, and research arenas. Dietetic technicians must complete a two-year associate degree in an ADA-approved dietetic technician program and then pass the registration examination for dietetic technicians. Dietary managers complete a one-year college course.

Effective teamwork requires shared goals, clearly defined roles, and a plan for coordinating efforts. Whenever possible, the patient should be part of the team. Any health professional can testify to the importance of patient cooperation in the diagnostic, therapeutic, and rehabilitative processes.

SUGGESTED ACTIVITIES

1. Contact a large medical center or hospital in your area to see if a dietetic team is present. Talk to the members of the team to determine their roles and responsibilities in delivering nutritional care to clients.

2. With a team of fellow students, write a paper on the principles of teamwork. In doing the research and writing the paper, apply the principles that have been found to be effective. Evaluate your success as a team. What worked well and why? What didn't work and why?

3. Choose any of the allied health professions. Do an in-depth study of its educational requirements, job responsibilities, areas of specialization, and so on.

4. Visit a local hospital cafeteria, and talk to as many of its employees as you can. Try to determine if, how, and to what extent they work with members of the dietetic team.

5. Volunteer to work in a hospital or other healthcare facility. This is an excellent way to learn about various healthcare professions and help those who need it at the same time.

NOTES

1. Balch GI. Employers' perceptions of the roles of dietetics practitioners: Challenges to survive and opportunities to thrive. *Journal of the American Dietetic Association*, 1996;96:1301–1305.

2. JIST Works, Inc. *America's Top 300 Jobs*. 6th ed. Indianapolis: JIST Works, Inc., 1998.

3. Shedlock N. Prognosis for careers in health: Never better. *Journal of Career Planning and Employment*, 1992;52:37–40.

4. Torrens PR. *The American Health Care System: Issues and Problems*. St. Louis, Mo.: C.V. Mosby Company, 1978.

5. Pellegrino ED. Interdisciplinary education in the health professions. In: *Educating for the Health Team*. Washington, D.C.: National Academy of Sciences, National Institute of Medicine, 1972. Allen AS, ed. *Introduction to Health Professions*. St. Louis, Mo.: C.V. Mosby Company, 1983.

6. Etzweiler DD. The patient is a member of the medical team. *Journal of the American Dietetic Association*, 1972;61:421–423.

7. Modrow CL, Darnell RE. Cross-modality: Delivery of health services through nonprofessionals. *Journal of the American Dietetic Association*, 1979;74:337–340. Modrow CL, Darnell RE. Dietetic services in cross-modality systems. *Journal of the American Dietetic Association*, 1979;74:341–344.

8. Tobias AL, Gordon JB. Social consequences of obesity. *Journal of the American Dietetic Association*, 1980;76:338–342.

PART THREE

Preparing for Practice

CHAPTER 4

Education and Training

One of the first actions of the fledgling American Dietetic Association (ADA) was the establishment of a teaching section, to provide guidance in the education and training of dietitians.[1] Through the years, the ADA has continued to be mindful of the education of future professionals, modifying educational standards to meet the ever-changing needs of the marketplace.

Two major study commissions, one in 1972 and another in 1984, were formed to make recommendations regarding the many questions facing dietetic education.[2] Other task forces, such as the Task Force on Education in 1982, the Critical Issues Task Force in 1992, and the Dietetic Education Task Force in 1993, have also addressed issues of importance to the educational process.[3]

What knowledge, skills, and abilities are necessary for successful dietetics practice? Should there be dietetic specialties? What kind of preparation is necessary for specialization? Should dietetic education programs be approved or accredited? How are entry-level practice and advanced practice different? The questions could go on and on: Dietetic education programs are always evolving as the profession of dietetics continues to change and grow.

THE COMMISSION ON ACCREDITATION/APPROVAL FOR DIETETICS EDUCATION

The Commission on Accreditation/Approval for Dietetics Education (CAADE) is recognized as the accrediting agency for associate degree dietetic technician programs, baccalaureate and graduate-level coordinated programs in dietetics, and post-baccalaureate dietetic internships. CAADE is also the accrediting agency for didactic programs in dietetics. CAADE exists to serve the public by establishing and enforcing standards for the educational preparation of dietetics professionals. They also recognize dietetic education programs that meet these standards.[4]

The Commission consists of ten individuals:

The chair

The chair-elect

The chair of the Review Panel for Coordinated Programs

The chairs of the two Review Panels for Didactic Programs in Dietetics

The chairs of the two Review Panels for Dietetic Internships

The chair of the Review Panel for Dietetic Technician Programs

Two representatives of the public

All of the members of the commission are elected by the general ADA membership with the exception of the two representatives of the public. The CAADE chair appoints these individuals.

The review panels are composed of both educators and practitioners who are responsible for reviewing programs based on the policies and procedures developed by CAADE. All CAADE members must have a minimum of a master's degree, be registered dietitians, and have at least five years of experience in dietetics education or practice.[5]

A BRIEF HISTORY OF DIETETIC EDUCATION REQUIREMENTS

In 1923, dietetic educators first outlined the courses they believed were necessary to prepare a student for dietetics practice. In 1927, the ADA approved the "Outline for Standard Course for Student Dietitians in Hospitals." This document required that students have a baccalaureate degree with a major in foods and nutrition and at least six months of training in a hospital (Figure 4.1) under the direction of a dietitian. The first list of hospitals offering this approved course was published in 1928.

In 1947, the academic expectations for students entering internships were published and became known as Plan I. Plan II, which covered four subject areas with a range of semester hours, was introduced in 1955. Plan III, begun in 1958, approached the educational process by designating core subjects, emphases, and concentrations. Plan IV, which included competency-based minimum academic requirements, was published in 1971. In 1987, Plan V was implemented, with *Knowledge Requirements for Dietitians*. Plan V also

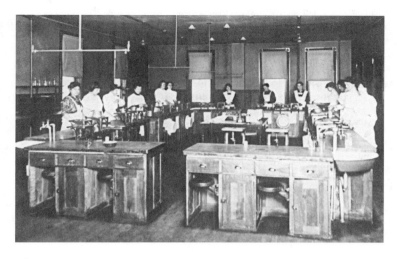

Figure 4.1
A very early food science laboratory.

Photo courtesy of The American Dietetic Association.

specified *Performance Requirements for Entry-Level Dietitians* to describe the skills that must be demonstrated or performed by those completing the supervised practice component of a dietetic education program. In 1987, the Council on Education of the ADA voted to discontinue the numbering of its educational plans. The *Standards of Education* were introduced as the minimum criteria to be met by all dietetic education programs. The latest version of the *Standards of Education* has been published in the fourth edition of *The Accreditation/Approval Manual for Dietetics Education Programs* by CAADE[6] in 1997 (Figures 4.2 through 4.6).

For many years, the only way to become a dietitian was to complete a postbaccalaureate dietetic internship. However, in 1962 the first Coordinated Undergraduate Program in Dietetics was developed. This type of program combined the required internship with the academic program. The student's hands-on experiences were coordinated with what was being discussed in the classroom, with the goal of making this combined learning experience even more meaningful. Through the Coordinated Undergraduate Program, a student could fulfill the academic and experience requirements in four years rather than five.

In the early 1970s, the need for dietetic support personnel led to the development of associate degree programs for dietetic technicians. These programs combined a two-year associate degree with 450 hours of hands-on experience. In 1974, guidelines for approving dietetic technician programs were introduced. In the 1980s, Approved

The entry-level dietitian is knowledgeable in the eight areas listed below. The foundation knowledge and skills precede achievement of the core and emphasis area(s) competencies, which identify the performance level expected upon completion of the supervised practice program.

Foundation learning is divided as follows: basic knowledge of a topic, working or in-depth knowledge of a topic as it applies to the profession of dietetics, and ability to demonstrate the skill at a level that can be developed further. To successfully achieve the foundation knowledge and skills, graduates must have demonstrated the ability to communicate and collaborate, solve problems, and apply critical thinking skills.

A. COMMUNICATIONS
   Graduates will have *basic knowledge about:*
   A.1.1. Negotiation techniques
   A.1.2. Lay and technical writing
   A.1.3. Media presentations
   Graduates will have *working knowledge of:*
   A.2.1. Interpersonal communications skills
   A.2.2. Counseling theory and methods
   A.2.3. Interviewing techniques
   A.2.4. Educational theory and techniques
   A.2.5. Concepts of human and group dynamics
   A.2.6. Public speaking
   A.2.7. Educational materials development
   Graduates will have *demonstrated the ability to:*
   A.3.1. Present an educational session for a group
   A.3.2. Counsel individuals on nutrition
   A.3.3. Demonstrate a variety of documentation methods
   A.3.4. Explain a public policy position regarding dietetics
   A.3.5. Use current information technologies
   A.3.6. Work effectively as a team member
B. PHYSICAL AND BIOLOGICAL SCIENCES
   Graduates will have *basic knowledge about:*
   B.1.1. Exercise physiology
   Graduates will have *working knowledge of:*
   B.2.1. Organic chemistry
   B.2.2. Biochemistry
   B.2.3. Physiology
   B.2.4. Microbiology
   B.2.5. Nutrient metabolism
   B.2.6. Pathophysiology related to nutrition care
   B.2.7. Fluid and electrolyte requirements
   B.2.8. Pharmacology: Nutrient-nutrient and drug-nutrient interaction

Figure 4.2
Foundation knowledge and skills for didactic component of entry-level dietitian education programs.

Graduates will have *demonstrated the ability to:*
B.3.1.   Interpret medical terminology
B.3.2.   Interpret laboratory parameters relating to nutrition
B.3.3.   Apply microbiological and chemical considerations to process controls

C.   SOCIAL SCIENCES
Graduates will have *basic knowledge of:*
C.1.1.   Public policy development
Graduates will have *working knowledge of:*
C.2.1.   Psychology
C.2.2.   Health behaviors and educational needs
C.2.3.   Economics and nutrition

D.   RESEARCH
Graduates will have *basic knowledge of:*
D.1.1.   Research methodologies
D.1.2.   Needs assessments
D.1.3.   Outcomes-based research
Graduates will have *working knowledge of:*
D.2.1.   Scientific method
D.2.2.   Quality improvement methods
Graduates will have *demonstrated ability to:*
D.3.1.   Interpret current research
D.3.2.   Interpret basic statistics

E.   FOOD
Graduates will have *basic knowledge of:*
E.1.1.   Food technology
E.1.2.   Biotechnology
E.1.3.   Culinary techniques
Graduates will have *working knowledge of:*
E.2.1.   Sociocultural and ethnic food consumption issues and trends for various consumers
E.2.2.   Food safety and sanitation
E.2.3.   Food delivery systems
E.2.4.   Food and non-food procurement
E.2.5.   Availability of nutrition programs in the community
E.2.6.   Formulation of local, state, and national food security policy
E.2.7.   Food production systems
E.2.8.   Environmental issues related to food
E.2.9.   Role of food in promotion of a healthy lifestyle
E.2.10. Promotion of pleasurable eating
E.2.11. Food and nutrition laws/regulations/policies
E.2.12. Food availability and access for the individual, family, and community
E.2.13. Applied sensory evaluation of food

Graduates will have *demonstrated the ability to:*

E.3.1. Calculate and interpret nutrient composition of foods
E.3.2. Translate nutrition needs into menus for individuals and groups
E.3.3. Determine recipe/formula proportions and modifications for volume food production
E.3.4. Write specifications for food and foodservice equipment
E.3.5. Apply food science knowledge to functions of ingredients in food
E.3.6. Demonstrate basic food preparation and presentation skills
E.3.7. Modify recipe/formula for individual or group dietary needs

F. NUTRITION

Graduates will have *basic knowledge of:*

F.1.1. Alternative nutrition and herbal therapies
F.1.2. Evolving methods of assessing health status

Graduates will have *working knowledge of:*

F.2.1. Influence of age, growth, and normal development on nutritional requirements
F.2.2. Nutrition and metabolism
F.2.3. Assessment and treatment of nutritional health risks
F.2.4. Medical nutrition therapy, including alternative feeding modalities, chronic diseases, dental health, mental health, and eating disorders
F.2.5. Strategies to assess need for adaptive feeding techniques and equipment
F.2.6. Health promotion and disease prevention theories and guidelines
F.2.7. Influence of socioeconomic, cultural, and psychological factors on food and nutrition behavior

Graduates will have *demonstrated ability to:*

F.3.1. Calculate and/or define diets for common conditions, i.e., health conditions addressed by health promotion/disease prevention activities or chronic diseases of the general population, e.g., hypertension, obesity, diabetes, diverticular disease
F.3.2. Screen individuals for nutritional risk
F.3.3. Collect pertinent information for comprehensive nutrition assessments
F.3.4. Determine nutrient requirements across the lifespan, i.e., infants through geriatrics and a diversity of people, culture, and religions
F.3.5. Measure, calculate, and interpret body composition data
F.3.6. Calculate enteral and parenteral nutrition formulas

G. MANAGEMENT

Graduates will have *basic knowledge about:*

G.1.1. Program planning, monitoring, and evaluation
G.1.2. Strategic management
G.1.3. Facility management
G.1.4. Organizational change theory
G.1.5. Risk management

Figure 4.2
continued

Graduates will have *working knowledge of:*
G.2.1. Management theories
G.2.2. Human resource management, including labor relations
G.2.3. Materials management
G.2.4. Financial management, including accounting principles
G.2.5. Quality improvement
G.2.6. Information management
G.2.7. Systems theory
G.2.8. Marketing theory and techniques
G.2.9. Diversity issues
Graduates will have *demonstrated the ability to:*
G.3.1. Determine costs of services/operation
G.3.2. Prepare a budget
G.3.3. Interpret financial data
G.3.4. Apply marketing principles
H. HEALTH CARE SYSTEMS
Graduates will have *basic knowledge about:*
H.1.1. Health care policy and administration
H.1.2. Health care delivery systems
Graduates will have *working knowledge of:*
H.2.1. Current reimbursement issues
H.2.2. Ethics of care

Source: Commission on Accreditation/Approval for Dietetics Education (CAADE), The American Dietetic Association. *Accreditation/Approval Manual for Dietetics Education Programs.* 4th ed. Chicago, Ill.: The American Dietetic Association, 1997. Reprinted with permission.

Competency statements specify what every dietitian should be able to do at the beginning of his or her practice career. The core competency statements build on appropriate knowledge and skills necessary for the entry-level practitioner to perform reliably at the verb level indicated. One or more of the emphasis areas should be added to the core competencies so that a supervised practice program can prepare graduates for identified market needs. Thus, all entry-level dietitians will have the core competencies and additional competencies according to the emphasis area(s)completed.

The minimum performance level for the competency is indicated by the action verb used at the beginning of the statement. The action verbs reflect four levels of performance. The higher level of performance assumes the ability to perform at the lower level:

1. *assist*—independent performance under supervision, or *participate*—take part in team activities;

2. *perform*—able to initiate activities without direct supervision, or *conduct*—activities performed independently;

3. *consult*—able to perform specialized functions that are discrete delegated activities intended to improve the work of others, or *supervise*—able to oversee daily operation of a unit including personnel, resource utilization, and environmental issues, or coordinate and direct the activities of a team or project workgroup;

4. *manage*—able to plan, organize, and direct an organization unit through actual or simulated experiences, including knowing what questions to ask.

If the verb "manage" is used, it assumes that the student will progress from "supervise" or "perform/do" the activity while in the program. (Note: the perform level is indicated in parentheses at the end of the statements to which it applies.) Students may demonstrate that they can manage or supervise through such activities as quality improvement audits, systems review, or directing an activity coordinating others.

Core Competencies for Dietitians (CD)

Upon completion of the supervised practice component of dietitian education, all graduates will be able to do the following:

CD1. Perform ethically in accordance with the values of The American Dietetic Association
CD2. Refer clients/patients to other dietetics professionals or disciplines when a situation is beyond one's level or area of competence (perform)
CD3. Participate in professional activities
CD4. Perform self-assessment and participate in professional development.
CD5. Participate in legislative and public policy processes as they affect food, food security, and nutrition
CD6. Use current technologies for information and communication activities (perform)
CD7. Supervise documentation of nutrition assessment and interventions

Figure 4.3
Competency statements for the supervised practice component of entry-level dietitian education programs.

CD8. Provide dietetics education in supervised practice settings (perform)

CD9. Supervise counseling, education, and/or other interventions in health promotion/disease prevention for patients/clients needing medical nutrition therapy for common conditions, e.g., hypertension, obesity, diabetes, and diverticular disease

CD10. Supervise education and training for target groups

CD11. Develop and review educational materials for target populations (perform)

CD12. Participate in the use of mass media for community-based food and nutrition programs

CD13. Interpret and incorporate new scientific knowledge into practice (perform)

CD14. Supervise quality improvement, including systems and customer satisfaction, for dietetics service and/or practice

CD15. Develop and measure outcomes for food and nutrition services and practice (perform)

CD16. Participate in organizational change and planning and goal-setting processes

CD17. Participate in business or operating plan development

CD18. Supervise the collection and processing of financial data

CD19. Perform marketing functions

CD20. Participate in human resources functions

CD21. Participate in facility management, including equipment selection and design/redesign of work units

CD22. Supervise the integration of financial, human, physical, and material resources and services

CD23. Supervise production of food that meets nutrition guidelines, cost parameters, and consumer acceptance

CD24. Supervise the development and/or modification of recipes/formulas

CD25. Supervise translation of nutrition into foods/menus for target populations

CD26. Supervise design of menus as indicated by patient's/client's health status

CD27. Participate in sensory evaluation of food and nutrition products

CD28. Supervise procurement, distribution, and service within delivery systems

CD29. Manage safety and sanitation issues related to food and nutrition

CD30. Supervise nutrition screening of individual patients/clients

CD31. Supervise nutrition assessment of individual patients/clients with common medical conditions, e.g., hypertension, obesity, diabetes, diverticular disease

CD32. Assess nutritional status of individual patients/clients with complex medical conditions, i.e., more complicated health conditions in select populations, e.g., renal disease, multi-system organ failure, trauma

CD33. Manage the normal nutrition needs of individuals across the lifespan, i.e., infants through geriatrics and a diversity of people, cultures, and religions

CD34. Design and implement nutrition care plans as indicated by the patient's/client's health status (perform)

CD35. Manage monitoring of patients'/clients' food and/or nutrient intake
CD36. Select, implement, and evaluate standard enteral and parenteral nutrition regimens, i.e., in a medically stable patient to meet nutritional requirements where recommendations/adjustments involve primarily macronutrients (perform)
CD37. Develop and implement transitional feeding plans, i.e., conversion from one form of nutrition support to another, e.g., total parenteral nutrition to tube feeding to oral diet (perform)
CD38. Coordinate and modify nutrition care activities among caregivers (perform)
CD39. Conduct nutrition care component of interdisciplinary team conferences to discuss patient/client treatment and discharge planning
CD40. Refer patients/clients to appropriate community services for general health and nutrition needs and to other primary care providers as appropriate (perform)
CD41. Conduct general health assessment, e.g. blood pressure, vital signs (perform)
CD42. Supervise screening of the nutritional status of the population and/or community groups
CD43. Conduct assessment of the nutritional status of the population and/or community groups
CD44. Provide nutrition care for population groups across the lifespan, i.e., infants through geriatrics, and a diversity of people, cultures, and religions (perform)
CD45. Conduct community-based health promotion/disease prevention programs
CD46. Participate in community-based food and nutrition program development and evaluation
CD47. Supervise community-based food and nutrition programs

Figure 4.3
continued

Source: Commission on Accreditation/Approval for Dietetics Education (CAADE), The American Dietetic Association. Accreditation/Approval Manual for Dietetics Education Programs. 4th ed. Chicago, Ill.: The American Dietetic Association, 1997. Reprinted with permission.

The core competencies ensure that everyone enrolled in a coordinated program or dietetic internship program has learning experiences reflecting the breadth of dietetics practice. The core provides the broad base of diverse experiences necessary for future career mobility.

All dietetic education supervised practice programs must offer at least one emphasis area. The emphasis areas are not intended to prepare specialists or advanced level practitioners as defined for credentialing purposes. Competencies for each emphasis area build on the core competencies and are designed to begin to develop the depth necessary for future proficiency in that area of dietetics practice. More experience in at least one area provides a model for learning throughout one's professional life.

For establishing an emphasis area, the program has the following options:

- Use one or more of the four defined emphasis areas; or,
- Develop a general emphasis by selecting a minimum of seven competency statements, relevant to program mission and goals, with at least one from each of the four defined emphasis areas. The selected competencies should build on the core competencies. General emphasis does not mean achievement of all competencies from all emphasis areas; or,
- Create a unique emphasis with a minimum of seven competency statements, based on environmental resources and identified needs.

Four emphasis areas and corresponding competencies for each emphasis are identified below.

Nutrition Therapy Emphasis Competencies (NT)

NT1. Supervise nutrition assessment of individual patients/clients with complex medical conditions, i.e., more complicated health conditions in select populations, e.g., renal disease, multi-system organ failure, trauma

NT2. Integrate pathophysiology into medical nutrition therapy recommendations (perform)

NT3. Supervise design through evaluation of nutrition care plans for patients/clients with complex medical conditions, i.e., more complicated health conditions in select populations, e.g., renal disease, multi-system organ failure, trauma

NT4. Select, monitor, and evaluate complex enteral and parenteral nutrition regimes, i.e., more complicated health conditions in select populations, e.g., renal disease, multi-system organ failure, trauma

NT5. Supervise development and implementation of transition feeding plans from the inpatient to the home setting

NT6. Conduct counseling and education for clients/patients with complex needs, i.e., more complicated health conditions in select populations, e.g., renal disease, multi-system organ failure, trauma

NT7. Perform basic physical assessment

NT8. Participate in nasoenteric feeding tube placement and care

NT9. Participate in waivered point-of-care testing, such as blood glucose monitoring

Figure 4.4
Competency statements for entry-level dietitian education programs emphasis areas.

NT10. Participate in the care of patients/clients requiring adaptive feeding devices

NT11. Manage clinical nutrition services

Community Emphasis Competencies (CO)

CO1. Manage nutrition care for population groups across the lifespan

CO2. Conduct community-based food and nutrition program outcome assessment/evaluation

CO3. Develop community-based food and nutrition programs (perform)

CO4. Participate in nutrition surveillance and monitoring of communities

CO5. Participate in community-based research

CO6. Participate in food and nutrition policy development and evaluation based on community needs and resources

CO7. Consult with organizations regarding food access for target populations

CO8. Develop a health promotion/disease prevention intervention project (perform)

CO9. Participate in waivered point-of-care testing, such as hematocrit and cholesterol levels

Foodservice Systems Management Emphasis Competencies (FS)

FS1. Manage development and/or modification of recipes/formulas

FS2. Manage menu development for target populations

FS3. Manage applied sensory evaluation of food and nutrition products

FS4. Manage production of food that meets nutrition guidelines, cost parameters, and consumer acceptance

FS5. Manage procurement, distribution, and service within delivery systems

FS6. Manage the integration of financial, human, physical, and material resources

FS7. Manage safety and sanitation issues related to food and nutrition

FS8. Supervise customer satisfaction systems for dietetics services and/or practice

FS9. Supervise marketing functions

FS10. Supervise human resource functions

FS11. Perform operations analysis

Business/Entrepreneur Emphasis Competencies (BE)

BE1. Perform organizational and strategic planning

BE2. Develop business or operating plan (perform)

BE3. Supervise procurement of resources

BE4. Manage the integration of financial, human, physical, and material resources

BE5. Supervise organizational change process

BE6. Supervise coordination of services

BE7. Supervise marketing functions

Figure 4.4
continued

Source: Commission on Accreditation/Approval for Dietetics Education (CAADE), The American Dietetic Association. *Accreditation/Approval Manual for Dietetics Education Programs.* 4th ed. Chicago, Ill.: The American Dietetic Association, 1997. Reprinted with permission.

The entry-level dietetic technician is knowledgeable in the eight areas listed below. The foundation knowledge and skills may be integrated with achievement of the competencies, which identify the performance level expected upon completion of the supervised practice component of the program.

Foundation learning is divided as follows: basic knowledge of a topic, working or in-depth knowledge of a topic as it applies to the profession of dietetics, and ability to demonstrate the skill at a level that can be developed further. To successfully achieve the foundation knowledge and skills, graduates must have demonstrated the ability to communicate and collaborate, solve problems, and apply critical thinking skills.

A. COMMUNICATIONS
Graduates will have *basic knowledge about:*
A.1.1.   Counseling theory and methods
A.1.2.   Methods of teaching
A.1.3.   Concepts of human and group dynamics
A.1.4.   Educational materials development
Graduates will have *working knowledge of:*
A.2.1.   Interpersonal communication skills
A.2.2.   Interviewing techniques
A.2.3.   Basic mathematics
A.2.4.   Written communication
Graduates will have *demonstrated the ability to:*
A.3.1.   Present an educational session for target groups
A.3.2.   Counsel individuals on nutrition for common conditions, i.e., health conditions addressed by health promotion/disease prevention activities or chronic diseases of the general population, e.g., hypertension, obesity, diabetes, diverticular disease
A.3.3.   Speak in front of a group
A.3.4.   Demonstrate a variety of documentation methods
A.3.5.   Use current information technologies
A.3.6.   Work effectively as a team member

B. PHYSICAL AND BIOLOGICAL SCIENCES
Graduates will have *basic knowledge about:*
B.1.1.   Applied concepts of chemistry
B.1.2.   Applied concepts of physiology
B.1.3.   Applied concepts of microbiology
B.1.4.   Nutrient-nutrient and drug-nutrient interactions
Graduates will have *demonstrated ability to:*
B.2.1.   Interpret medical terminology
B.2.2.   Interpret laboratory parameters relating to nutrition
B.2.3.   Apply microbiological and chemical consideratios to recipe development

C. SOCIAL SCIENCES
Graduates will have *basic knowledge about:*
C.1.1.   Psychology/sociology

Figure 4.5
Foundation knowledge and skills for didactic component of entry-level dietetic technician education programs.

C.1.2.   Health behaviors and educational needs
C.1.3.   Economics and nutrition
C.1.4.   Public policy issues
D.   RESEARCH
Graduates will have *basic knowledge about:*
D.1.1.   Interpretation of current research
D.1.2.   Needs assessment
D.1.3.   Basic statistics
D.1.4.   Quality improvement
E.   FOOD
Graduates will have *basic knowledge about:*
E.1.1.   Sociocultural and ethnic food consumption issues and trends for various consumers
E.1.2.   Food technology issues
E.1.3.   Availability of nutrition programs in the community
E.1.4.   Environmental issues related to food
E.1.5.   Promotion of pleasurable eating
E.1.6.   Food availability and access for the individual, the family, and the community
E.1.7.   Food and nutrition laws/regulations/policies
E.1.8.   Role of food in promotion of a healthy lifestyle
Graduates will have *working knowledge of:*
E.2.1.   Basic concepts and techniques of food preparation
E.2.2.   Applied sensory evaluation of food
E.2.3.   Food production systems
E.2.4.   Food delivery systems
E.2.5.   Food and non-food procurement
Graduates will have *demonstrated the ability to:*
E.3.1.   Calculate and analyze nutrient composition of foods
E.3.2.   Translate nutrition needs into menus for individuals and groups
E.3.3.   Determine recipe/formula proportions and modifications for volume food production
E.3.4.   Apply functions of ingredients in food preparation
E.3.5.   Write specifications for food and equipment
E.3.6.   Assist with food demonstrations
E.3.7.   Apply food safety and sanitation techniques
F.   NUTRITION
Graduates will have *basic knowledge about:*
F.1.1.   Fundamentals of nutrition and metabolism
F.1.2.   Assessment of health risks
F.1.3.   Influence of socioeconomic, cultural, and psychological factors on food and nutrition behavior
F.1.4.   Health promotion and disease prevention theories
F.1.5.   Strategies to assess need for adaptive feeding techniques and equipment

Figure 4.5
continued

Graduates will have *working knowledge of:*
F.2.1.   Influence of age, growth, and normal development on nutrition requirements
F.2.2.   Applied clinical nutrition
Graduates will have *demonstrated the ability to:*
F.3.1.   Calculate diets for common conditions, i.e. health conditions addressed by health promotion/disease prevention activities or chronic diseases of the general population, e.g., hypertension, obesity, diabetes, diverticular disease
F.3.2.   Screen individuals for nutritional risk
F.3.3.   Determine nutrient requirements across the lifespan, i.e., infants through geriatrics and a diversity of people, culture, and religions
F.3.4.   Measure and calculate body composition
F.3.5.   Calculate basic enteral and parenteral nutrition formulas

G.   MANAGEMENT
Graduates will have *basic knowledge about:*
G.1.1.   Program planning, monitoring, and evaluation
G.1.2.   Marketing theory and techniques
G.1.3.   Systems theory
G.1.4.   Labor relations
G.1.5.   Materials management
G.1.6.   Financial management
G.1.7.   Facility management
G.1.8.   Quality improvement
G.1.9.   Risk management
G.1.10. Diversity issues
Graduates will have *working knowledge of:*
G.2.1.   Applied management theories
G.2.2.   Applied human resources management
G.2.3.   Information management
Graduates will have *demonstrated the ability to:*
G.3.1.   Collect and interpret information
G.3.2.   Determine costs of services/operations

H.   HEALTH CARE SYSTEMS
Graduates will have *basic knowledge about:*
H.1.1.   Current reimbursement issues
H.1.2.   Health care policy
H.1.3.   Health care delivery systems
Graduates will have *working knowledge of:*
H.2.1.   Ethics of care

Source: Commission on Accreditation/Approval for Dietetics Education (CAADE), The American Dietetic Association. *Accreditation/Approval Manual for Dietetics Education Programs.* 4th ed. Chicago, Ill.: The American Dietetic Association, 1997. Reprinted with permission.

Competency statements specify what every dietetic technician should be able to do at the beginning of his or her practice career. The competency statements build on appropriate knowledge and skills necessary for the entry-level practitioner to perform reliably at the level indicated.

The minimum performance level for the competency is indicated by the action verb used at the beginning of the statement. The action verbs reflect four levels of performance. The higher level of performance assumes the ability to perform at the lower level:

1. *assist*—independent performance under supervision, or *participate*—take part in team activities;

2. *perform*—able to initiate activities without direct supervision, or *conduct*—activities performed independently;

3. *consult*—able to perform specialized functions that are discrete delegated activities intended to improve the work of others, or *supervise*—able to oversee daily operation of a unit including personnel, resource utilization, and environmental issues, or coordinate and direct the activities of a team or project workgroup;

4. *manage*—able to plan, organize, and direct an organization unit through actual or simulated experiences, including knowing what questions to ask.

If the verb "supervise" is used, it assumes that the graduate will progress from "perform/do" the activity while in the program. (Note: the perform level is indicated in parenthesis at the end of the statements to which it applies.) Students may demonstrate that they can supervise an activity rather than an individual, through such activities as quality improvement audits or coordinating the work of others.

Competencies for Dietetic Technicians (DT)

Upon completion of the supervised practice component of a dietetic technician education program, the graduate will be able to do the following:

DT1. Perform ethically in accordance with the values of The American Dietetic Association

DT2. Refer clients/patients to other dietetics professionals or disciplines when a situation is beyond one's level of competence (perform)

DT3. Participate in professional activities

DT4. Perform self-assessment and participate in professional development

DT5. Participate in legislative and public policy processes as they affect food, food security, and nutrition

DT6. Use current technologies for information and communication activities (perform)

DT7. Document nutrition screenings, assessments, and interventions (perform)

DT8. Provide dietetics education in supervised practice settings (perform)

DT9. Educate patients/clients in disease prevention and health promotion and medical nutrition therapy for common conditions, e.g., hypertension, obesity, diabetes, diverticular disease (perform)

Figure 4.6

Competency statements for the supervised practice component of entry-level dietetic technician education programs.

DT10. Conduct education and training for target groups

DT11. Assist with development and review of educational materials for target populations

DT12. Apply new knowledge or skills to practice (perform)

DT13. Participate in quality improvement, including systems and customer satisfaction, for dietetics service and/or practice

DT14. Participate in development and measurement of outcomes for food and nutrition services and practice

DT15. Participate in organizational change and planning and goal setting processes

DT16. Participate in development of departmental budget/operational plan

DT17. Collect and process financial data (perform)

DT18. Assist with marketing functions

DT19. Participate in human resources functions

DT20. Participate in facility management, including equipment selection and design/redesign of work units

DT21. Supervise organizational unit, including financial, human, physical, and material resources and services

DT22. Supervise production of food that meets nutrition guidelines, cost parameters, and consumer acceptance

DT23. Develop and/or modify recipes/formulas (perform)

DT24. Supervise translation of nutrition into foods/menus for target populations

DT25. Design menus as indicated by the patient's/client's health status (perform)

DT26. Participate in applied sensory evaluation of food and nutrition products

DT27. Supervise procurement, distribution, and service within delivery systems

DT28. Supervise safety and sanitation issues

DT29. Perform nutrition screening of individual patients/clients

DT30. Assess nutritional status of individual patients/clients with common medical conditions, i.e., health conditions addressed by health promotion/ disease prevention activities or chronic diseases of the general population, e.g. hypertension, obesity, diabetes, diverticular disease (perform)

DT31. Assist with nutrition assessment of individual patients/clients with complex medical conditions, i.e., more complicated health conditions in select populations, e.g., renal disease, multi-system organ failure, trauma

DT32. Participate in the management of the normal nutrition needs of individuals across the lifespan, i.e., infants through geriatrics and a diversity of people, cultures, and religions

DT33. Assist with design and implementation of nutrition care plans as indicated by the patient's/client's health status

DT34. Monitor patients'/clients' food and/or nutrient intake (perform)

DT35. Participate in the selection, monitoring, and evaluation of standard enteral nutrition regimes, i.e., in a medically stable patient to meet nutritional requirements where recommendations/adjustments involve primarily macronutrients

DT36. Implement transition feeding plans (perform)

DT37. Participate in interdisciplinary team conferences to discuss patient/client treatment and discharge planning

DT38. Refer patients/clients to appropriate community services for general health and nutrition needs and to other primary care providers as appropriate (perform)

DT39. Conduct general health assessment, e.g., blood pressure, vital signs

DT40. Conduct screening of the nutritional status of the population and/or community groups

DT41. Assist with assessment of the nutritional status of the population and/or community groups

DT42. Participate in nutrition care for population groups across the lifespan, i.e., infants through geriatrics and a diversity of people, cultures, and religions

DT43. Participate in community-based or worksite health promotion/disease prevention programs

DT44. Participate in development and evaluation of community-based food and nutrition programs

DT45. Implement and maintain community-based food and nutrition programs (perform)

Figure 4.6
continued

Source: Commission on Accreditation/Approval for Dietetics Education (CAADE), The American Dietetic Association. *Accreditation/Approval Manual for Dietetics Education Programs.* 4th ed. Chicago, Ill.: The American Dietetic Association, 1997. Reprinted with permission.

Pre-Professional Practice Programs, known as AP4s, were developed. These postbaccalaureate programs were similar to dietetic internships but provided some new features. AP4s were introduced as a means of encouraging the sponsorship of dietetic education programs by non-traditional dietetic practice settings such as business and industry, public health departments, or school districts. The AP4s enabled students to complete program requirements through part-time work.

In 1993, the Dietetic Education Task Force recommended that all postbaccalaureate supervised practice programs would become known as *internships* and their participants as *interns*. Thus, the distinction between AP4s and dietetic internships will be eliminated in the years ahead, reducing the confusion that surrounds the two types of post-baccalaureate supervised practice programs. Another change is that all dietetic programs, including dietetic technician programs and didactic programs in dietetics, now must be accredited rather than approved, and undergo a site visit by CAADE.

CAADE'S STANDARDS OF EDUCATION AND THE ACCREDITATION/APPROVAL PROCESS

The CAADE's Standards of Education outline five prerequisites that must be met by every dietetic education program:

1. The mission statement or philosophy and measurable goals for the program shall provide guidance to the program.
2. Fair, equitable, and considerate treatment of both prospective students and those enrolled in an educational program will be incorporated into all aspects of the program.
3. Resources available to the program shall be identified and their contribution to the program described.
4. The curriculum shall provide for attainment of the expected competence of the program graduate.
5. A systematic approach shall be used in managing and evaluating the program.

Before a dietetic program can begin accepting students, the program's director and faculty members must undertake an in-depth review process known as a *self-study*. The process for conducting a self-study is outlined in CAADE's *Accreditation/Approval Manual for*

Dietetic Education Programs.[7] The self-study document outlines in detail how the dietetic program meets the ADA Standards of Education. The written self-study document is then forwarded to the appropriate CAADE review panel.

A dietetic education program that offers only the coursework necessary to meet the *Foundation Knowledge and Skills for the Didactic Component of Entry-Level Dietitian Education Programs* (Figure 4.2) is called a *didactic program in dietetics (DPD)*. After this program submits a self-study that acceptably demonstrates how it meets the five Standards of Education, the program becomes an *approved* dietetic education program, meaning that it passed a pencil-and-paper review by the CAADE. As of December 1998, DPDs must become accredited through a site visit, in addition to the self-study. During the site visit, representatives of the CAADE actually visit the dietetics program.

Since coordinated programs and dietetic technician programs provide both the academic component and the supervised practice component, the self-study for these programs must outline how they meet both the *Foundation Knowledge and Skills for the Didactic Component* (see Figures 4.2 and 4.5) and the *Competency Statements for the Supervised Practice Component* (see Figures 4.3 and 4.6) for their respective types of programs.[8] Once the pencil-and-paper review of the self-study document is completed by the CAADE Review Panel, two or three site visitors are dispatched to visit the program and verify that what was presented in the self-study document is actually occurring. The site visit is a required step for all programs with a supervised practice component seeking to be accredited by the CAADE. The pencil-and-paper review and the site visit assure students, parents, administrators, and others that the dietetic education program meets the high standards set by the CAADE of the ADA.

GRIEVANCE/COMPLAINT PROCEDURE

If any individual, such as a student, faculty member, dietetics practitioner, or member of the public, has a complaint about any accredited/approved dietetics education program, they may submit a complaint or grievance to CAADE. All written grievances are forwarded to the Chair of CAADE for action. According to CAADE, the Commission

> will not intervene on behalf of individuals or act as a court of appeal for individuals in matters of admissions, appointment, promotion, or dismissal or faculty or students. It will intervene only when it determines that the practices or conditions indicate that the program may not be in compliance with the Standards of Education or with published accreditation/approval guidelines.[9]

P R O F I L E

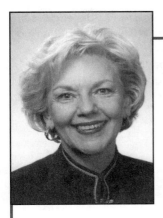

Stella Cash, M.Ed., M.S., R.D.

POSITION
> Program Director of Dietetics and Senior Academic Specialist, Michigan State University, East Lansing, MI

EDUCATION
> B.S. University of Central Arkansas, Conway, AR
> M.Ed. University of Arkansas, Fayetteville, AR
> M.S. Michigan State University, East Lansing, MI

ROUTE TO REGISTRATION
> Master's plus experience

When I graduated in the mid-1960s, it was difficult for a married woman to receive a dietetic internship appointment, and if you had children, you could just forget about it! Thankfully, the profession has changed since then! Because I couldn't become a registered dietitian (R.D.) at the time, I taught high school biology and chemistry for 12 years early in my career. When I came to Michigan State University in 1975, I was appointed to a half-time position advising dietetics students. Soon after that, I learned I could use my master's degree plus a six-month planned work experience to become eligible to sit for the R.D. exam. Thus, I became an R.D.

◆ **Professional Involvement**
President, Michigan Dietetic Association
Delegate to ADA's House of Delegates for eight years
First Chair of the Council on Professional Issues
ADA-PAC Committee
Weekly television show for 1½ years

◆ **Honors and Awards Received**
1997 ADA Medallion Award
Michigan State University, College of Human Ecology Outstanding Teaching Award
Michigan State University, College of Human Ecology Advising/Professional Mentoring Award
Recipient of Outstanding Alumni Award, University of Central Arkansas
Michigan Dietetic Association's highest award

◆ **Words of Wisdom for Future Dietetics Professionals**
Working with hundreds of dietetic students over the past 25 years, I have been able to observe the characteristics of many successful indi-

viduals. I have also seen a revolution in the profession of dietetics: job market shifts, the recognition of the critical role of food to nutrition and health, and the impact of technology.

Based on my experience, observations, and the projected trends, the successful new-millennium dietitian will need:

√ Strong management and communication skills
√ Research-based competency
√ Willingness to take risk
√ Twenty-first-century technology skills
√ Involvement in the political arena
√ Passion for your job

Michigan State University has provided me the opportunity to travel extensively to many parts of the world and to use my consultant time working with food companies and the restaurant industry. This background has given me real-world working knowledge to share in the classroom.

The profession of dietetics offers many opportunities for leadership development and career advancement. Dietetics has no boundaries, and only you will set the limits!

THE THREE STEPS TO BECOMING A REGISTERED DIETITIAN OR DIETETIC TECHNICIAN, REGISTERED

There are three components in the preparation for dietetics practice: education, supervised practice, and credentialing. These three steps apply whether you wish to become a dietetic technician, registered (D.T.R.) or a registered dietitian (R.D.).

To become a D.T.R., you must

1. Complete a two-year associate degree in an accredited dietetic technician program that meets the *Foundation Knowledge and Skills for the Didactic Component of Entry-Level Dietetic Technician Education Programs*[10] (see Figure 4.5) as outlined by the CAADE.

2. Complete a minimum of 450 hours of supervised practice experience that meets the *Competency Statements for the Supervised Practice Component of Entry-Level Dietetic Technician Education Programs*[11] (see Figure 4.6). This experience must be gained under the direction of an accredited dietetic technician program.

3. Successfully complete the national Registration Examination for Dietetic Technicians.

To become an R.D., you must

1. Complete a baccalaureate degree in an accredited didactic program in dietetics or an accredited coordinated program in dietetics that meets the *Foundation Knowledge and Skills for the Didactic Component of Entry-Level Dietitian Education Programs*[12] (see Figure 4.2), as outlined by the CAADE.
2. Complete a minimum of 900 hours of supervised practice experience within an accredited coordinated program or in an accredited dietetic internship that meets the *Competency Statements for the Supervised Practice Component of Entry-Level Dietitian Education Programs*[13] (see Figure 4.3).
3. Successfully complete the national Registration Examination for Dietitians.

THE ACADEMIC EXPERIENCE

The academic preparation to become a dietitian may be obtained in either an accredited didactic program or a coordinated program in dietetics. Dietetic technician students obtain their academic preparation in an accredited dietetic technician program. The dietetics curriculum may be slightly different at different universities, because each school has unique strengths and resources. Graduates of DPDs are eligible to apply for postbaccalaureate supervised practice programs to meet ADA's requirements. Graduates of a coordinated program in dietetics meet *both* academic and supervised practice requirements in their degree programs and are eligible to sit for the Registration Examination for Dietitians on completion of their program. Likewise, graduates of an accredited dietetic technician program meet *both* academic and supervised practice requirements in their associates degree program and are eligible to sit for the Registration Examination for Dietetic Technicians on completion of their program.

A typical dietetics curriculum might include courses such as written communications, speech, psychology, sociology, economics, and humanities courses. Courses in biology, anatomy and physiology, microbiology, chemistry, organic chemistry, and biochemistry are also required. Support courses often include organization and management, accounting, marketing, educational theory, or other courses. Professional courses might include normal nutrition, clinical nutrition, public health nutrition, food science, quantity food production, and

foodservice purchasing. Students who are participating in a coordinated program in dietetics or a dietetic technician program also will
have courses that have a supervised practice component.

The *Directory of Dietetics Programs 1998–1999*[14] lists 230 didactic programs approved by the ADA. As these programs complete their
next self-study process, they will also undergo a site visit to become
accredited programs. There are didactic programs in dietetics in the
District of Columbia, Puerto Rico, and all states except Alaska. Some
states have numerous programs: Texas has 17, California, 16 and Illinois, 11 approved programs. Currently, 49 coordinated programs in
dietetics, 218 dietetic internships, and 70 dietetic technician programs
are accredited by CAADE.

Students seeking admission to supervised practice programs
should realize that grade-point average, particularly in the physical
and biological sciences, is an important criteria for acceptance. Many
supervised practice programs look for applicants with at least a 3.0
grade-point average (on a 4.0-scale) to be considered for appointment.
A solid academic base is essential for success in a supervised practice
experience. Other criteria critical to success in obtaining a supervised
practice experience include dietetics-related work experience in a variety of dietetics practice settings, volunteer experience in the community, and demonstrated leadership ability.

THE SUPERVISED PRACTICE EXPERIENCE

CAADE requires a minimum of 900 hours of supervised practice experience for registration-eligibility as a dietitian, which may be obtained
in a coordinated program or dietetic internship, or 450 hours for registration-eligibility as a dietetic technician in a dietetic technician program. A dietetic internship is a postbaccalaureate experience for graduates of didactic programs and may include graduate coursework as
well as the supervised practice experience. Graduates of a coordinated
program or a dietetic technician program have already completed
supervised practice experience.

Supervised practice experience may be either full-time (40 hours
per week) or part-time (20 hours per week). However, the program
must be specifically designed with a part-time component for the student to use this approach. Supervised practice in a coordinated program in dietetics may vary from a few hours per week at the junior
level to 30 to 35 hours per week at the senior level. Students in coordinated programs and in dietetic technicians programs are also taking
didactic coursework along with their supervised practice experience.

Most supervised practice experiences are unpaid, although some
postbaccalaureate experiences do provide a stipend. The *Directory of*

Dietetics Programs 1998–1999[15] provides information on stipends, length of programs, number of students accepted per class, and other important information. The Dietetic Educators of Practitioners Practice Group (DEP) also produces a publication entitled *The Applicant Guide to Supervised Practice Programs,*[16] which is an excellent resource for students comparing the requirements of different programs. Check with your program director to see if your university has a copy of this guide for your use.

Some postbaccalaureate supervised practice programs combine the opportunity to earn graduate credits or complete a master's degree with the supervised practice experience. Some programs *require* a master's degree in conjunction with the practical experience; other programs make completion of the graduate degree optional. Students applying for these programs must meet the graduate-school requirements of the institution to which they are applying. Typically, a minimum grade-point average of 3.0 is required. Many programs also require that the applicant submit scores from the Graduate Records Examination (GRE) as part of the supervised practice program application. Applicants should contact the program director to obtain information on a specific supervised practice program.

Students applying for dietetic internships may apply to as many different programs around the United States as they wish. However, participation in a computer matching process is also required. Students are asked to fill out a computer mark-sense card that forces them to rank order their preferences of the programs to which they have applied. The computer-matching program then compares each applicant's rank-ordered list of programs she or he is interested in with supervised practice programs' rank-ordered list of individuals they would like to see in their program. When a match is found, the student is notified for acceptance or rejection of the placement. It is recommended that students apply to more than one program in order to increase their chances of placement for the supervised practice experience.

Supervised practice experiences are based on the *Competency Statements for the Supervised Practice Component of Entry-Level Dietitian Education Programs* (see Figure 4.3) or *of Entry-Level Dietetic Technician Programs* (see Figure 4.6).[17] Supervised practice programs, like their didactic counterparts, are designed to take advantage of the strengths and expertise of each program's faculty and staff. All supervised practice programs provide experiences in nutrition services delivery, community nutrition or public health nutrition, and foodservice systems management, although the amount of time spent in each of these areas varies from program to program. ADA does not mandate equal emphasis in the three areas but does expect that all areas will be covered in the supervised practice program.

The supervised practice experience is one of the most meaningful parts of preparation for dietetics practice. The opportunity to work alongside practicing dietetic professionals is exciting and challenging, and the hands-on experiences bring the information presented during the academic program to life. Thus, the supervised practice experience is an important step in helping students move from theory to the reality of dietetic practice.

Supervised practice experiences are designed to move from simple to complex, from functioning with assistance to functioning alone, from student to entry-level dietitian or entry-level dietetic technician. Frequently, a student will observe a task being performed by a dietitian or dietetic technician. Next, the student will attempt the activity with guidance from the professional. Finally, the student progresses to independent functioning. At each step, students are evaluated, and specific feedback is provided to enhance the learning experience. Early experiences may involve role playing or other forms of simulation so students can develop skills in a low-risk environment. As skill levels and confidence increase, the student is allowed to take on more and more responsibility. Culminating experiences, such as "staff relief," allow the student to function independently as a full-fledged dietitian or dietetic technician and, thus, give the student a realistic picture of dietetics practice.

VERIFICATION OF EDUCATION AND SUPERVISED PRACTICE EXPERIENCE

On successful completion of the education and supervised practice components, the student is issued a verification statement. This form is a legal document and should be treated as such. This document, bearing the original signature of the program director, verifies that the student successfully completed the education and/or supervised practice experience. Students completing a DPD and a postbaccalaureate supervised practice program will have two verification statements; students completing a coordinated program will have only one form. These statements must be presented when the student changes from associate to active membership in the ADA or when the graduate applies for a license to practice dietetics in a state that has licensure for dietitians.

Students enrolled in a dietetic technician program must also present a verification statement before sitting for the national Registration Examination for Dietetic Technicians. Since dietetic technician programs combine education with supervised practice, only one verification statement is issued on program completion.

SUMMARY

Preparation for entry into the profession of dietetics encompasses both prescribed academic preparation and supervised hands-on experience. Both of these components are carefully structured and monitored by the ADA through its Council on Professional Issues and the Commission on Accreditation/Approval for Dietetics Education. Ongoing role delineation studies form the basis for the *Foundation Knowledge and Skills* (see Figures 4.2 and 4.5) and the *Competency Statements* (see Figures 4.3, 4.4, and 4.6) used to guide the development of both academic curricula and supervised practice experiences.[18]

The challenge facing ADA and dietetic educators is to keep educational preparation on the cutting edge of professional practice, ensuring that current students will be prepared for the exciting future that awaits them as dietetic technicians and registered dietitians. The most important focus must be on the development of critical thinking and problem-solving skills, so future dietitians know HOW to think, rather than WHAT to think. You must be prepared to take responsibility for your own continued professional development, since information about food and nutrition issues is expanding at an exponential rate. Learn how to learn, and you will be ready for an exciting future in dietetics.

SUGGESTED ACTIVITIES

1. Find out about the history of your dietetics program. When did the program begin? How many people have graduated from your program? What are some of those graduates doing now?

2. Interview a dietitian in your area. Find out the following information:

    a. How did you learn about the profession of dietetics?
    b. What kind of dietetics education program did you go through?
    c. What was your first dietetics position?
    d. What other dietetics positions have you held?
    e. Describe your current job and its responsibilities.
    f. What skills do you believe are necessary for successful dietetics practice?
    g. What do you like best about being a dietitian or dietetic technician?

3. Obtain a copy of the *Directory of Dietetics Programs*[19] from your program director. Are there other dietetics education programs in your state? in a neighboring state? If so, where are they? What

kinds of programs are offered? Contact some of the students in these programs and network with them.

NOTES

1. Cassell J. *Carry the Flame: The History of the American Dietetic Association*. Chicago, Ill.: The American Dietetic Association, 1990.

2. *The Profession of Dietetics: The Report of the Study Commission on Dietetics*. Chicago, Ill.: The American Dietetic Association, 1972.

3. Haschke MB, Maize RS. President's Page: Dietetic education: The future and policy decisions. *Journal of The American Dietetic Association*, 1984;84:208–212.

4. Commission on Accreditation/Approval for Dietetics Education (CAADE). *Achieving Excellence in Dietetics Education*. Brochure developed by CAADE/The American Dietetic Association, 1997.

5. Ibid.

6. Commission on Accreditation/Approval for Dietetics Education (CAADE), The American Dietetic Association. *Accreditation/Approval Manual for Dietetics Education Programs*. 4th ed. Chicago, Ill.: The American Dietetic Association, 1997.

7. Ibid.

8. Ibid.

9. CAADE. *Achieving Excellence*.

10. CAADE, ADA. *Accreditation/Approval Manual*.

11. Ibid.

12. Ibid.

13. Ibid.

14. The American Dietetics Association. *Directory of Dietetics Programs 1998–1999*. Chicago, Ill.: The American Dietetic Association, 1998.

15. Ibid.

16. Dietetics Educators of Practitioners Practice Group. *The Applicant Guide to Supervised Practice Programs—1997–98*. Chicago, Ill.: Dietetics Educators of Practitioners Practice Group, 1999.

17. CAADE, ADA. *Accreditation/Approval Manual*.

18. Ibid.

19. ADA. *Directory of Dietetics Programs 1998–1999*.

CHAPTER 5

◆

Credentialing

Defining the competence required of practitioners is an important quality-assurance activity for any profession. According to Webster's, the word *credential* means "a letter or certificate given to a person to show that he has a right to confidence or to the exercise of a certain position or authority; that which gives credit; that which entitles to credit, confidence, etc., establishing reliability."[1] This is an appropriate description of the work of the Commission on Dietetic Registration (CDR).

THE COMMISSION ON DIETETIC REGISTRATION

CDR, the credentialing arm of the American Dietetic Association (ADA), was first called the Committee on Professional Registration. In 1969, it was charged with the implementation of dietetic registration. In November 1975, CDR was made an independent unit of the ADA. CDR is responsible for all aspects of the registration process: standard setting for registration eligibility, examination development and administration, credentialing, and recertification. CDR grants recognition of entry-level competence to dietitians who meet its standards and qualifications. These dietitians may use the legally protected professional designation *Registered Dietitian* or the initials *R.D.* Dietetic technicians who meet the standards and qualifications for technicians may use the legally protected professional designation *Dietetic Technician, Registered* or the initials *D.T.R.*

CDR was originally made up of eight persons elected by the ADA membership. In 1979, a public member, who represents users of the services of R.D.s and D.T.R.s, was added to the Commission. In 1990, a D.T.R. representative became a member of CDR, to represent the interests of dietetic technicians. In 1994, a CDR-certified specialist was appointed to the Commission. In 1995, a Fellow of the ADA representative was added to the Commission. In all, the CDR comprises 12 members.[2]

DIETETIC REGISTRATION

The purpose of registration is to protect the nutritional health, safety, and welfare of the public by encouraging high standards of performance of persons practicing in the profession of dietetics.[3] Registration of dietitians began in 1969, providing a legally protected title for credentialed practitioners. At its inception, registration required membership in the ADA, completion of an examination, and a continuing education requirement. More than 19,000 members of the ADA became registered during the initial enrollment period, when the examination was waived.[4] Currently, there are 63,557 R.D.s.[5] Membership in the ADA is no longer a requirement for R.D. status.

The role of the dietetic technician is not to be overlooked. Dietetic technicians were first admitted to membership in the ADA in 1975. Certification for Dietetic Technicians Registered (D.T.R.) became a reality in 1983. CDR currently recognizes 5,372 D.T.R.s.[6]

THE REGISTRATION EXAMINATION

The development of the examinations for R.D. and D.T.R. status is rigorous. Figure 5.1 outlines the steps in CDR's test development program. *Role delineation* is the important first step in this process. A role delineation study is an in-depth research study with the goal of describing the knowledge and skills necessary to competently practice dietetics at a specified level (in this instance, entry level). Because the role delineation study surveys current practitioners in the field, using it as a basis for test development ensures that the certification test is job related, representative of current practice, and geared to the appropriate level of responsibility.

From the role delineation study, a blueprint for building the examination must be developed. *Test specifications* include a description of what is to be tested, the proportion of the test to be devoted to various content areas, and the characteristics of acceptable test items. Because the test specifications come from the role delineation study, the test is valid and credible.

Test item development is an exciting but time-consuming experience. Test questions are developed by individuals trained in the specifics of test construction. Care is taken in choosing individuals who represent a diversity of practice, geographic, and ethnic backgrounds. Four criteria are applied to each test question: (1) the question must be relevant and critical to entry-level practice; (2) the ques-

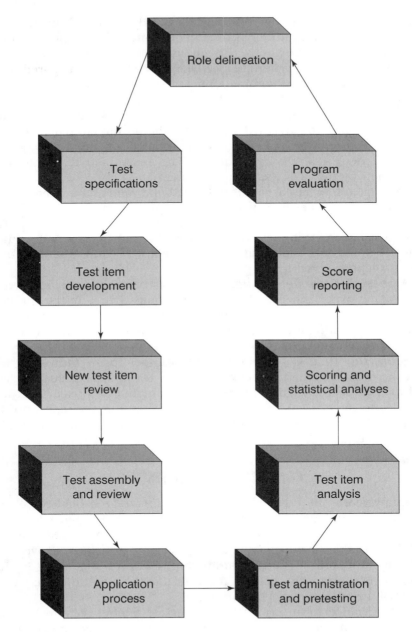

Figure 5.1
Certification testing program.

Reprinted with permission, Commission on Dietetic Registration. The American Dietetic Association, Chicago, Ill.

tion must be accurate, current, and clear; (3) the question must not reflect regional or institutional differences; and (4) the question must conform to test specifications. Test items are reviewed by professional test editors and item writers before being pretested as unscored items on actual administered examinations.

During the *test assembly and review* process, a draft test is assembled from items in the computerized test bank. Experienced test reviewers appointed by CDR review the items for content accuracy, currency, and relevance to entry-level practice. They must also be sure that each item has one best answer. The assembled test undergoes final review by the CDR Examination Panel.

After each test has been administered and items have been scored, psychometricians perform *test item analysis*. Performance statistics are reviewed for each test question to identify any problems. Test items that appear to be problematic are reviewed by experienced item writers before score reporting, to eliminate any questions with ambiguities or response errors.

A *passing-score determination study* is periodically conducted by CDR, using experienced dietetics professionals from diverse practice areas and population subgroups. This passing score becomes the basis for evaluating future examinations, to ensure that all versions of the test are of equal difficulty.

Score reporting is twofold. One report goes to the individual who took the examination. This report gives the test a total scaled score as well as raw scores in the different test domains or areas. CDR also provides to dietetic education programs both summary reports of the institution's graduates and individual scores if an examinee has authorized CDR to do so.[7]

COMPUTER ADAPTIVE TESTING

For many years, the R.D. and D.T.R. exams have been held twice each year, in April and October. These have been pencil-and-paper examinations administered in cooperation with American College Testing (ACT). Test takers have usually had to wait approximately six weeks to find out the results of their examination. However, beginning in July 1999, registration examinations for both dietitians and dietetic technicians will be administered by computer.

CDR decided to implement computerized testing because it recognized the many advantages this method offers to examinees. These include

- Flexible test administration dates; examinees can schedule testing throughout the year, rather than only twice a year.
- Retesting is available six weeks following the previous test date.

- Unique examination is based on each examinee's entry-level competence.
- Score reports are distributed to examinees as they leave the test site, eliminating the six-week waiting period required with pencil-and-paper testing.

The registration examinations will be administered at over two hundred approved test sites nationwide operated by the Sylvan Learning Corporation (Sylvan Learning Centers). Eligible candidates can call a Sylvan testing site to schedule an appointment to take their examination. Costs will be $125 for the *Registration Examination for Dietitians* and $80 for the *Registration Examination for Dietetic Technicians*.

The examinations will be variable in length. For the R.D. examination, each test taker will be given a *minimum* of 125 questions; 100 of these are scored questions, and 25 of these are questions that are being pretested for use on subsequent examinations and are unscored. The *maximum* number of questions possible is 145; 120 are scored questions, and 25 are unscored pretest questions.

For the technician examination, each examinee will be given a *minimum* of 110 questions; 80 of these are scored questions, and 30 are unscored pretest questions. The *maximum* number of questions is 130, with 100 being scored items and 30 being unscored pretest items. For both examinations, test takers are given three hours, which includes time for an introductory tutorial.

Students would be advised to practice taking a computerized test if they have never done so. On the computerized examination, the test taker is not allowed to change answers, skip questions, or review their responses. CDR has prepared an informational diskette that describes the computerized testing process. This diskette, entitled *Computer Adaptive Testing: A New World of Options in Assessment*, is available free of charge from CDR by calling (800) 877-1600, extension 5500. This diskette will also be included in all copies of the study guides provided by CDR for the examinations.[8]

Individuals who have completed both the academic preparation and supervised practice requirements and have received signed verification statements for both of these experiences may sit for the national Registration Examination for Dietitians or the Registration Examination for Dietetic Technicians. A verification statement signed by the program director and a transcript documenting completion of the required courses must be submitted with the examination application. If an individual is returning to college or university to complete a degree started at some earlier time, a dietetics program may require the individual to update previous coursework before issuing a verification statement to that individual. You should check with the dietetics program director to find out about such program requirements.

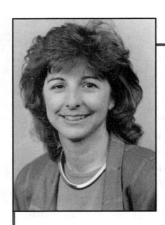

PROFILE

Cyndi Thomson, Ph.D., R.D., C.N.S.D., F.A.D.A.

POSITION
  Clinical Nutrition Research Specialist, Arizona Prevention Center, and Clinical Lecturer, Department of Medicine, University of Arizona, Tucson, AZ

EDUCATION
  B.S. West Virginia University, Morgantown, WV
  M.S. University of Arizona, Tucson, AZ
  Ph.D. University of Arizona, Tucson, AZ

ROUTE TO REGISTRATION
  Coordinated program in dietetics

◆ **Positions Held**
  Consultant for nutrition education materials development, Medical Directions, Inc., Tucson, AZ
  Chief Clinical Dietitian, University Medical Center, Tucson, AZ
  Senior Dietitian, Kino Community Hospital, Tucson, AZ
  Consultant, El Rio Neighborhood Health Center, HIV Early Intervention Nutrition Clinic, Tucson, AZ
  Clinical Nutrition Specialist, Nutrition Support in Critical Care, Oncology, Acquired Immune Deficiency Syndrome, General Medicine, Family Medicine, University Medical Center, Tucson, AZ
  Consultant Dietitian in Long-Term Care, Santa Rosa Convalescent Center, Tucson, AZ
  Adjunct Faculty, Central Arizona College Dietetic Education Program

◆ **Professional Involvement**
  Chair, Nutrition Educators of Health Care Professionals Practice Group of the ADA
  Executive Board, Arizona Society of Parenteral and Enteral Nutrition
  Delegate from Arizona to ADA's House of Delegates
  President, Southern Arizona Dietetic Association
  Media spokesperson for the ADA on phytochemicals and functional foods
  Members of ADA's expert review panel for publication of dietary supplement use

◆ **Honors and Awards Received**
  Award of Merit, Arizona Dietetic Association
  Dietitian of the Year, University Medical Center, Tucson
  Recognized Young Dietitian of the Year, Arizona

◆ **Words of Wisdom for Future Dietetics Professionals**
Dietetics is a wonderful profession. The world is full of opportunities. No longer is the R.D. relegated to clinical practice. R.D.s can move into research, the food industry, private counseling, health and fitness, journalism—the potential areas of practice are limited only by your own imagination. And if the decision is to practice in the clinical realm, it is bound to be rewarding as dietitians gain more and more autonomy and respect from healthcare providers.

Be imaginative, creative, flexible, and assertive, and you will have a rewarding and fulfilling career. Remember, "the world is your oyster"— or your apple or maybe even mango! As nutrition research and knowledge expand, the R.D. will be integral to translating the information obtained into practical and effective lifestyle changes for Americans and others worldwide.

Dietetics has afforded me the opportunity to challenge my intellect, develop strong professional partnerships, do something meaningful that serves others, and to have a balanced life.

MAINTAINING REGISTERED STATUS

Continuing education has always been an integral part of professional registration. As the profession of dietetics continues to change and expand into new areas of practice, it is vital that dietetics professionals be lifelong learners. As we move into new and uncharted waters, each of us must update and broaden our knowledge base for effective dietetics practice. CDR was one of the first health credentialing agencies to insist on continuing education. To maintain registered status, dietetics professionals must document their participation in professional development activities by creating a Professional Development Portfolio. R.D.s must achieve seventy-five Continuing Professional Education Units (CPEUs), and D.T.R.s must achieve fifty CPEUs during each five-year reporting period. The CPEUs must be based on each person's individual learning needs as identified in the professional development portfolio process.

PROFESSIONAL DEVELOPMENT PORTFOLIO STEPS

The steps in developing one's portfolio follow:

- Reflect on your professional practice in order to establish professional goals.

- Conduct a learning needs assessment to identify what you know and what you need to learn to reach your goals.
- Develop a learning plan that shows how you will meet your goals.
- Implement your learning plan through continuing professional development activities.
- Evaluate your learning plan outcomes to assess how you have applied what you've learned and its impact on reaching your goals, refocusing those goals when necessary.

CDR defines continuing education as education beyond that required for entry into the profession. Educational programs may apply directly to the field of nutrition and dietetics or may launch the learner into new areas such as computer technology, physical assessment, or marketing. Whatever the learning activity, it should update or enhance one's knowledge and skills for new applications in dietetics practice. Some examples of continuing education activities include

- Lectures
- Workshops
- Journal clubs and study groups
- Seminars
- Case presentations
- Video, audio, and computer-based materials
- Self-study programs
- Culinary skills training
- Physical assessment training
- Multiskilling training
- Computer-technology training[9]

CDR SELF-ASSESSMENT MODULES

In 1992, CDR made available the first of its self-assessment modules. Self-assessment is a method of continuing professional education that focuses on identifying strengths and needs. The series of modules developed by CDR are designed to help individual practitioners identify their learning needs, make well-informed decisions about how to spend their continuing education time and money, and design a continuing education action plan based on the individual's assessment results.

The modules may be completed at work or at home. They are self-paced, practice-oriented, and approved by CDR for continuing education credits. Modules may include videotape simulation exercises, print materials, case scenarios, or other tools. Questions assess the user's understanding of the concepts and problems presented. After completing a module, it is returned to be scored. An individual report is generated and mailed to the module user. Results are totally confidential and available only to the individual dietetic practitioner. The report provides an overall score and a comparison of the module user's score with others' scores, including the scores of other dietetics professionals who share significant professional characteristics. Information on how experts would answer each question and why is also provided. Finally, an action plan worksheet is provided to help the user to map future continuing education goals. Resources for further information on the subject matter are also included.

Some of the module topics include management, nutrition assessment, nutrition planning, nutrition implementation, nutrition evaluation, nutrition counseling, nutrition programs for consumers, managing financial resources, marketing new products, and conducting research. Other modules are scheduled for production in the years ahead.[10]

LICENSURE

Licensure is "a state policy that provides consumers an assurance that a professional is competent to provide certain services and is used by professionals to exclude the non-licensed from providing those services for a fee. It is a tool for creating and maintaining a verifiable minimum level of skill and competence."[11]

Licensure differs from registration in several ways. While registration is recognized nationally, licensure is recognition by an individual state. Both credentialing systems afford some legal protection to the title of the practitioner, but licensure may also protect the right of an individual to practice in a state. Registration is voluntary, established and maintained in the private sector. Licensure may be either voluntary or mandatory but has formal legal status in the public sector.

At the present time, 39 states, the District of Columbia, and Puerto Rico have enacted some form of regulation. *Licensing statutes* make it illegal to practice dietetics without first obtaining a license from the state. *Statutory certification* limits the use of particular titles to persons meeting predetermined requirements, but persons not certified can still practice dietetics with a different title. *Registration* is the least restrictive form of state regulation. It prohibits use of the title *dietitian* by persons not meeting state-mandated qualifications. However, unregistered persons may practice the profession.

Each state has a licensure contact person who can provide updates on professional regulation in that state. For the name and telephone number of any state's licensure contact, call the ADA at (202) 371-0500.

SPECIALTY CERTIFICATION

In 1993, the CDR first offered registered dietitians the opportunity to become board-certified specialists in different dietetic specialties. The current areas of dietetic specialization are renal nutrition and pediatric nutrition.

To become a board-certified specialist, one must document the following minimum criteria:

- Current registration status and three years minimum length of registration
- 6,000 hours of practice as a registered dietitian in the specialty over the last six years, and current employment of a minimum of 16 hours a week in the specialty area
- Successful completion of a practice certification examination

New areas of specialization may be recognized in the coming years. Specialty credentials are also available from other professional organizations. Some of these certifications follow:

- *Certified Nutrition Support Dietitian* by the National Board of Nutrition Support Certification, Inc., 8630 Fenton Street, Suite 412, Silver Spring, MD 20910. Phone: (301) 587-6315; Fax: (301) 587-2365; aspen@nutr.org.
- *Certified Lactation Consultant* by the International Board of Lactation Consultant Examiners, 7309 Arlington Boulevard, Suite 300, Falls Church, VA 22042. Phone: (703) 560-7330; Fax: (703) 560-7332; iblce@erols.com.
- *ACSM Certified Health/Fitness Instructor SM, ACSM Certified Health/Fitness Director, ACSM Certified Exercise Specialist,* or *ACSM Certified Program Director* by the American College of Sports Medicine, P.O. Box 1440, Indianapolis, IN 46206-1440. Phone: (317) 637-9200; Fax: (317) 634-7817; crtacsm@acsm.org.
- *Certified Health Education Specialist* by the National Commission for Health Education Credentialing, Inc., 944 Marcon Boulevard, Suite 310, Allentown, PA 18103. Phone: (888) 624-3248; Fax: (800) 813-0727; ncheccos@fast.net.
- *Certified Professional in Healthcare Quality* by the Healthcare Quality Certification Board, P.O. Box 1880, San Gabriel, CA 91778. Phone: (800) 346-4722; Fax: (626) 286-9415; www.cphq-hqcb.org.
- *National Certified Counselor* by the National Board for Certified Counselors, 3 Terrace Way, Suite D, Greensboro, NC 27403. Phone: (336) 547-0607; Fax: (336) 547-0017; www.nbcc.org.

- *School Food Service and Nutrition Specialist* by the American School Food Service Association, 1600 Duke Street, 7th Floor, Alexandria, VA 22314-3436. Phone: (703) 739-3900; Fax: (703) 739-3915; www.asfsa.org. (This is an approved certification for recertification of D.T.R.s only.)

Specialty credentials can be a valuable asset to the dietitian who holds them. Career advancement may be enhanced, salary levels may increase, and recognition of heightened expertise by other members of the healthcare team may be realized.

FELLOW OF THE AMERICAN DIETETIC ASSOCIATION

The ADA has established the credential of *fellow* to certify those registered dietitians who have demonstrated empirically defined characteristics of achievement and leadership. To become a fellow, candidates must fulfill the following requirements:

- Be a registered dietitian.
- Submit documentation of a minimum of a master's degree, earned and granted by a regionally accredited U.S. college or university or foreign equivalent.
- Submit documentation of a minimum of eight years' work experience as a registered dietitian.
- Submit documentation of at least one professional achievement.
- Submit documentation of professional positions.
- Submit documentation of professional contacts.
- Submit a written response to an approach-to-practice scenario.

A portfolio submitted by the candidate is judged through peer review. Certification as Fellow of The American Dietetic Association (FADA) is granted for a ten-year period. During that period, fellows are required to maintain R.D. status and submit an annual maintenance fee. At the end of the certification period, fellows who wish to recertify must submit an updated portfolio and a recertification fee.[12]

OTHER TOOLS SUPPORTING PROFESSIONAL COMPETENCE

The Standards of Professional Practice

The Standards of Professional Practice, revised in 1997 and published in the January 1998 issue of the *Journal of The American Dietetic*

Association, guide professional practice and encourage lifelong learning (see Chapter 6, Figure 6.11).

The Code of Ethics for the Profession of Dietetics

The Code of Ethics for the Profession of Dietetics is an enforceable code that provides for public accountability by monitoring appropriate ethical performance by a dietetics practitioner and reflects the individual's responsibility for competence in practice (see Chapter 6, Figure 6.12).

SUMMARY

Each of you should have the goal of becoming a credentialed dietetics practitioner. While completion of an associate or baccalaureate degree in dietetics is a worthy achievement, it is the earning of the professional credential of D.T.R. or R.D. that opens doors for successful professional practice. This credential is customers' assurance of your qualifications to practice, and it indicates that you actively work to update yourself on the latest information about food and nutrition issues. Licensure indicates that the state in which you practice recognizes your professional competence and expertise.

Specialty certification will become more common in the years ahead, as dietetics practice becomes increasingly complex and diverse. Recognition of leadership and exceptional practice in dietetics by attaining the Fellow of the ADA credential is a goal to which all students in dietetics should aspire. Professional credentialing is the mark of quality practice; it assures the public that the dietetic technician or registered dietitian is providing the highest quality in dietetics services.

SUGGESTED ACTIVITIES

1. Talk to someone who has recently taken the registration examination for dietitian or dietetic technician. What was their reaction to the experience? What suggestions do they have for preparing for the exam?

2. Who is your state continuing education coordinator? If possible, talk to this individual and find out what kinds of continuing education events he or she approves. What process must be followed to get an event approved for continuing education credit?

3. Attend a continuing education event with a dietetics professional, faculty member, or another student. What kind of documentation

must be provided for an attendee to receive continuing education credits?

4. Find out if your state has licensure for dietitians. If so, invite someone to your class to talk about licensure, what it means in your state, and how it was obtained in the legislature. What is the process for becoming licensed in your state?

NOTES

1. *Webster's New Universal Unabridged Dictionary*. 2nd ed. New York: Simon & Schuster, 1983.

2. Woodward NM. *The Past, Present, and Future of Dietetics Credentialing*. Future Search Conference: Challenging the Future of Dietetic Education and Credentialing. Background Papers. Chicago. Ill.: The American Dietetic Association and The Commission on Dietetic Registration, June 12–14, 1994.

3. Ibid.

4. Commission on Dietetic Registration of The American Dietetic Association, personal communication, October 1994.

5. Commission on Dietetic Registration of The American Dietetic Association, personal communication, November 1998.

6. Ibid.

7. *Components of the Certification Testing Program*. Chicago, Ill.: The Commission on Dietetic Registration, 1989.

8. *1998 Desk Reference for Educators*. Chicago, Ill.: Commission on Dietetic Registration, 1998.

9. *Professional Development Portfolio Guide*. Chicago, Ill.: Commission on Dietetic Registration, 1998.

10. *Self-Assessment: A New Approach to Continuing Professional Education*. Chicago, Ill.: Commission on Dietetic Registration, 1992.

11. Licensure of dietitians and nutritionists: Update on state laws. *Journal of The American Dietetic Association*, 1994;94:974.

12. *Fellow of the American Dietetic Association*. Chicago, Ill.: Commission on Dietetic Registration, 1998.

PART FOUR

Professional Associations

CHAPTER 6

Professionalism

What comes to mind when you hear someone described as professional? Responses to this question are generally varied and include such qualities as knowledgeable, ethical, caring, and well groomed. *Professionalism*, as defined by Webster's, is "the conduct, aims, or qualities that characterize or mark a profession or a professional person."[1] Along with the title *professional* comes a defined set of expectations. It is not enough to attain the title; one must also be committed to a well-defined pattern of responsibilities and activities.

In this chapter, we examine the conduct, aims, and qualities considered characteristic of the dietetics profession. We emphasize the importance of showing respect and concern for people, being knowledgeable and keeping current with the latest research in one's area of practice, adherence to the strictest ethical standards, and commitment to the profession. We also include the role of professional societies, the benefits of membership, and a description of a selection of societies in the field.

A HELPING PROFESSION

By its very nature, dietetics is a helping profession (Figure 6.1). Dietetic practice involves service to people.[2] The way this service is delivered is critically important. Respect, caring, and concern for people and their value systems are basic to the concept of professionalism. These characteristics may be manifested in many ways, not the least of which is respect for the dignity of each and every person. An understanding of individual differences—such as gender, ethnicity, and religion—is also critical for effective practice.

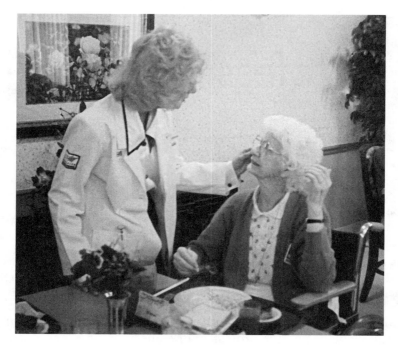

Figure 6.1
A dietary manager and one of her health center's
residents.

THE CHALLENGE AND REWARD OF LIFETIME LEARNING

Professional competence in the dietetic profession is ensured by the
autonomous credentialing body of The American Dietetic Association
(ADA), the Commission on Dietetic Registration. It requires that practitioners complete an approved or accredited educational program and
then maintain competence through a system of continuing education.
This continuing education may take the form of journal or textbook
reading or attending and participating in seminars, conferences, meetings, exhibits (Figures 6.2 and 6.3), and college courses (Figures 6.4
and 6.5). Because the field of nutrition is so dynamic, the form and
content of the continuing education should be carefully chosen to
enhance the quality of the professional's practice.

GOALS OF LIFETIME EDUCATION FOR THE DIETETIC PRACTITIONER

   1.   *Committed to excellence in the nutritional care of individuals and groups.*   All dietetic practitioners contribute to nutritional

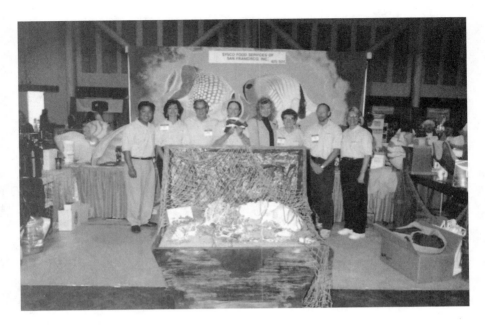

Figure 6.2
A major foodservice company exhibits at a state dietetic association annual meeting.

Source: California Dietetic Association. Reprinted with permission.

care. Dietetic practitioners are dedicated to excellence in professional service. In the pursuit of excellence, they are responsible for the establishment of goals and the assessment of progress towards these goals.

2. *Comprehend, interpret, and apply the science and art of nutrition in the promotion of individual, group, and community health.* Dietetic practitioners need a thorough knowledge of the scientific bases of human nutritional needs, including biochemical, physiological, and psychological relationships throughout life, in health and disease. Interpretation and application of the science of nutrition requires creativity in dealing with people and situations, knowledge of food in its many implications for health, and the ability to communicate directly to people or indirectly through the efforts of others for nutritional care.

3. *Understand the significance of scientific inquiry and interpretation in advancing professional knowledge and improving standards of performance.* It is essential for dietitians to understand and appreciate research and to be able to evaluate and interpret findings. The scope of dietetic research is broad. It includes such areas as

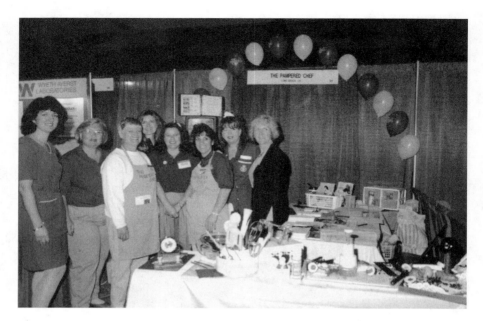

Figure 6.3
An entrepreneurial company exhibits at a state dietetic
association annual meeting.

Source: California Dietetic Association. Reprinted with permission.

nutritional (Figure 6.6), behavioral (Figure 6.7), and managerial sciences (Figure 6.8); technological developments in food production (Figures 6.9 and 6.10), processing, and marketing; foodservice systems
and equipment; and information processing. The dietetic practitioner
evaluates new research findings and uses those that are valid and
appropriate for the nutritional care of people.

   4. *Share responsibility with associated professionals by contributing specialized knowledge of nutrition.* Dietetic practitioners
collaborate with others in planning, executing, and evaluating comprehensive healthcare programs. The prevention, treatment, and control
of health problems of individuals, families, groups, or communities
often have a nutritional component. This care may be given in a variety
of settings: hospitals, extended-care facilities, government or voluntary
health agencies, industries, businesses, or schools.

   5. *Adapt planning and performance to environmental factors,
recognizing physiological, psychological, social, political, cultural,
and economic influences.* Dietetic practitioners are alert to emerging
concepts in science and technology, and the environmental influences

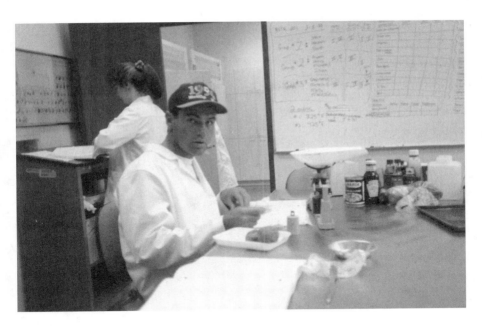

Figure 6.4
Students in a food science lab.

Source: Courtesy of Pepperdine University, Malibu, California.

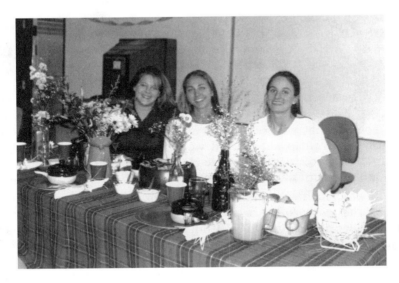

Figure 6.5
Students enjoy their term project in an introduction to foods class.

Source: Courtesy of Pepperdine University, Malibu, California.

Figure 6.6
A student conducting nutritional science research.

Source: Courtesy of Pepperdine University, Malibu, California.

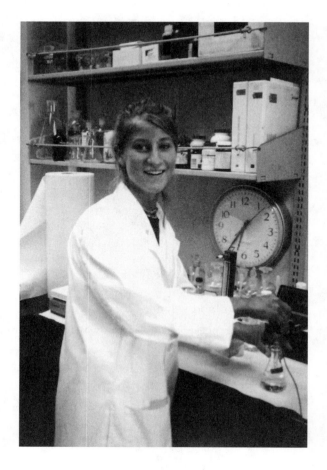

within society that will require alteration in order to achieve them. They are prepared to accept and work with individual differences in food practices and varying attitudes toward the role of nutrition in the promotion of health and the control of disease.

   6.   *Demonstrate respect and empathy for people and an appreciation of the individual's capacity to change and develop.*   Sensitivity to and acceptance of the attitudes and behavior of individuals is essential for teaching, guiding, and directing. Dietetic practitioners are responsible for providing an atmosphere in which an individual may be motivated to learn. When the teacher and the learner are mutually involved, both become better and more responsive individuals.

   7.   *Are competent in managing available resources in the provision of nutritional care.*   Management is the coordination of available resources to achieve specified goals. Managerial competency is essen-

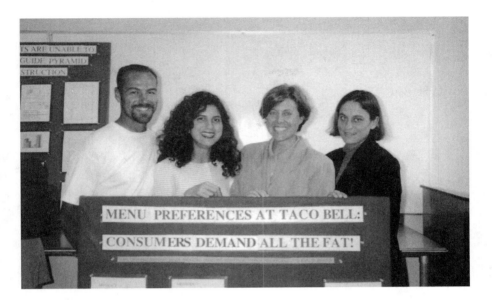

Figure 6.7
Students display their research projects.
Source: Courtesy of Pepperdine University, Malibu, California.

tial for all dietetic practitioners. The provision of nutritional care requires effective management of resources—physical facilities, finances, and people—so that people needing care receive it. New management theories and the evolution of healthcare emphasize the need for anticipatory management.

Dietetic practitioners recognize that one of their most important resources is themselves. Competency in management includes ability to assess and use one's own time and talents effectively.

8. *Manifest proficiency in communication.* Skill in communicating necessitates effective listening, speaking, reading, and writing. Dietetic practitioners, with an awareness of modern communication theory and methods, select the channels through which they can best communicate.

9. *Maintain the discipline and self-awareness of the professional and accept responsibility for their continuing professional development.* Recognition of the meaning of being professional—through self-appraisal, self-discipline, and continuing education—is essential for the dietetic practitioner. Planning for excellence necessitates formulating short- and long-term goals for professional development. Personal motivation, initiative, resourcefulness, and judgment need to be continuously exercised by the dietetic practitioner.

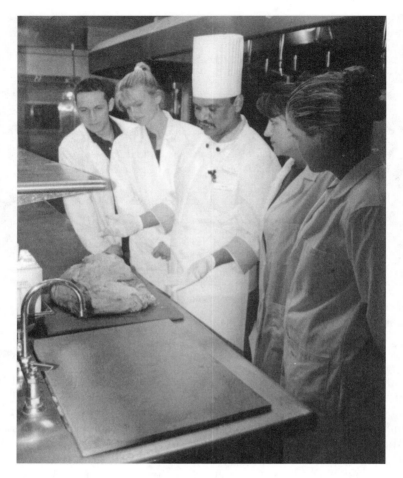

Figure 6.8
Dietetic interns discuss product procurement with a chef.

Source: Courtesy of Pepperdine University, Malibu, California.

Receptiveness to new experiences and the pursuit of scientific inquiry are integral to continuing development. With increasing breadth of experience comes increased self-confidence and potential. These attributes, together with increasing flexibility, will contribute immeasurably to a lifetime of creative productivity.[3]

Figure 6.9
A student experiments
on yeast dough.

Source: Courtesy of
Pepperdine University,
Malibu, California.

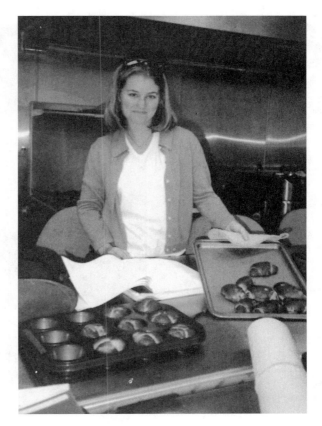

STANDARDS OF PRACTICE

The ADA House of Delegates adopted the current version of the Standards of Professional Practice in October 1997. These Standards outline a dietetic practitioner's responsibilities for providing quality nutritional care. The standards provide individual practitioners with a systematic plan for implementing, evaluating, and adjusting performance in any area of practice. The six Standards of Professional Practice, as shown in Figure 6.11, describe the key characteristics of the dietetic profession and focus on the results or outcomes of service.

Each standard is specifically defined by specific criteria. For example, Standard 6, Indicator 1 states, "Each dietetic professional conducts self-assessment at regular intervals to identify professional strengths and weaknesses."[4]

Figure 6.10
Student-conducted
experiment on yeast
dough.

Source: Courtesy of
Pepperdine University,
Malibu, California.

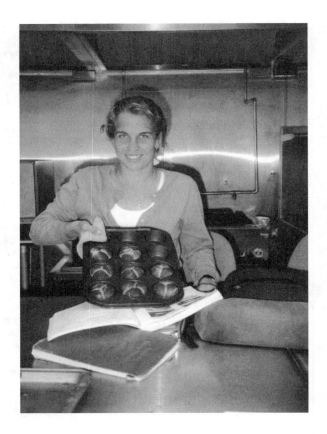

PROFESSIONAL ETHICS

Ethical issues faced by members of the dietetics profession are as
diverse as the settings in which members practice. In medical and clinical settings, patients' rights, confidentiality of information, and the
provision of food and water are the primary issues that must be con-
fronted. In foodservice settings, ethical issues revolve around the management of money, personnel, materials, and time. In research and
education, issues of plagiarism and research design involving animals
or human beings are issues of ethical concern.[5]

Every professional association must address the issue of acceptable professional behavior. This is usually accomplished through a
written document called a code of ethics. The code describes the philosophy and expectations of conduct to which the association agrees
its members should adhere. Figure 6.12 shows an example of one
such code of ethics, developed by The American Dietetic Association in
1987.[6]

STANDARD 1: PROVISION OF SERVICES

Develops, implements, and promotes quality service based on client expectations and needs

Rationale
Dietetics professionals provide, facilitate, and promote quality services based on client needs and expectations, current knowledge, and professional experience.

Indicators
Each dietetics professional:
1.1 collaborates with client to assess needs, background, and resources and to establish mutual goals
1.2 collaborates with other professionals as appropriate
1.3 applies knowledge and skills to determine the most appropriate action plan
1.4 implements quality practice by following policies, procedures, legislation, licensure, practice guidelines, and the Standards of Professional Practice
1.5 fosters excellence and exhibits professionalism in practice
1.6 continuously evaluates processes and outcomes
1.7 advocates for the provision of food and nutrition services as part of public policy

Examples of outcomes
- Clients actively participate in establishing goals and objectives
- Clients' needs are met
- Clients are satisfied with service and products provided
- Evaluation reflects expected outcomes
- Public has access to food and nutrition services

STANDARD 2: APPLICATION OF RESEARCH

Effectively applies, participates in or generates research to enhance practice

Rationale
Effective application, support, and generation of dietetics research in practice encourages continuous quality improvement and provides documented support for the benefit of the client.

Indicators
Each dietetics professional:
2.1 locates and reviews research findings for their application to dietetics practice
2.2 bases practice on sound scientific principles, research, and theory
2.3 promotes research through alliances and collaboration with dietetics and other professionals and organizations
2.4 contributes to the development of new knowledge and research in dietetics
2.5 collects measurable data and documents outcomes within the practice setting
2.6 shares research data and activities through various media

Figure 6.11
Standards 1 through 6 of the Standards of Professional
Practice developed by The American Dietetic Association.

Examples of outcomes
- Client receives appropriate services based on the effective application of research
- A foundation for performance measurement and improvement is provided
- Outcomes data supports reimbursement for the services of dietetics professionals
- Research findings are used for the development and revision of policies, procedures, practice guidelines, protocols, and clinical pathways
- Professionals use benchmarking and knowledge of "best practices" to improve performance

STANDARD 3: COMMUNICATION AND APPLICATION OF KNOWLEDGE

Successful dietetics professionals apply knowledge and communicate effectively with others

Rationale
Dietetics professionals work with and through others while using their unique knowledge of food, human nutrition, and management as well as skills in providing services.

Indicators
3.1 has knowledge related to a specific area(s) of professional service
3.2 communicates sound scientific principles, research, and theory
3.2 integrates knowledge of food and human nutrition with knowledge of health, social sciences, communication, and management theory
3.4 shares knowledge and information with clients
3.5 helps students and clients apply knowledge and skills
3.6 documents interpretation of relevant information and results of communication with professionals, personnel, students, or clients
3.7 contributes to the development of new knowledge
3.8 seeks out information to provide effective services

Examples of outcomes
- Professional provides expertise in food, nutrition, and management information
- Client understands the information received
- Clients receives current and appropriate information and knowledge
- Client knows how to obtain additional guidance

STANDARD 4: UTILIZATION AND MANAGEMENT OF RESOURCES

Uses resources effectively and efficiently in practice

Rationale
Appropriate use of time, money, facilities, and human resources facilitates delivery of quality services.

Figure 6.11
continued

Indicators

Each dietetics professional:

4.1 uses a systematic approach to maintain and manage professional resources successfully

4.2 uses measurable resources such as personnel, monies, equipment, guidelines, protocols, reference materials, and time in the provision of dietetics services

4.3 analyzes safety, effectiveness, and cost in planning and delivering services and products

4.4 justifies use of resources by documenting consistency with plan, continuous quality improvement, and desired outcome

4.5 educates and helps clients and others to identify and secure appropriate and available resources and services

Examples of outcomes

- The dietetics professional documents use of resources according to plan and budget
- Resources and services are measured and data are used to promote and validate the effectiveness of services
- Desired outcomes are achieved and documented
- Resources are managed and used cost-effectively

STANDARD 5: QUALITY IN PRACTICE

Systematically evaluates the quality and effectiveness of practice and revises practice as needed to incorporate the results of evaluation

Rationale

Quality practice requires regular performance evaluation and continuous improvement of services.

Indicators

Each dietetics professional:

5.1 identifies performance improvement criteria to monitor effectiveness of services

5.2 identifies expected outcomes

5.3 documents outcomes of services provided

5.4 compares actual performance to expected outcomes

5.5 documents action taken when discrepancies exist between actual performance and expected outcomes

5.6 continuously evaluates and refines services based on measured outcomes

Examples of outcomes

- Performance improvement criteria are measured
- Actual performance is evaluated
- Clients' outcomes meet established criteria (objectives/goals)
- Results of quality improvement activities and direct refinement of practice

STANDARD 6: CONTINUED COMPETENCE AND PROFESSIONAL ACCOUNTABILITY

Engaged in lifelong self-development to improve knowledge and skills that promote continued competence

Rationale

Professional practice requires continuous acquisition of knowledge and skill development to maintain accountability to the public.

Indicators

Each dietetics professional:

6.1 conducts self-assessment at regular intervals to identify professional strengths and weaknesses

6.2 identifies needs for professional development and mentors others

6.3 develops and implements a plan for professional growth

6.4 documents and professional development activities

6.5 adheres to the Code of Ethics for the profession of dietetics and is accountable and responsible for actions and behavior

6.6 supports the application of research findings to professional practice

6.7 takes active leadership roles

Examples of outcomes

- Dietetics professional uses self-reflection and feedback from a variety of sources to evaluate and implement professional change
- Dietetics professional development needs are identified and directed learning takes place
- Dietetics professional accepts accountability to the public
- Dietetics professional obtains appropriate certification
- Dietetics professional supports legislation which promotes positive food and nutrition outcomes
- Dietetics professional uses "best practices" to demonstrate competency
- Dietetics professional meets Commission on Dietetic Registration recertification requirements

Figure 6.11
continued

Source: The American Dietetic Association Standards of Professional Practice for Dietetics Professionals. Copyright The American Dietetic Association. Reprinted by permission from *JOURNAL OF THE AMERICAN DIETETIC ASSOCIATION,* Vol. 98:84–85, 1998.

Preamble

The American Dietetic Association and its credentialing agency, the Commission on Dietetic Registration, believe it is in the best interests of the profession and the public it serves that a *Code of Ethics* provide guidance to dietetic practitioners in their professional practice and conduct. Dietetic practitioners have voluntarily developed a *Code of Ethics* to reflect the ethical principles guiding the dietetic profession and to outline commitments and obligations of the dietetic practitioner to self, client, society, and the profession.

The purpose of the Commission on Dietetic Registration is to assist in protecting the nutritional health, safety, and welfare of the public by establishing and enforcing qualifications for dietetic registration and for issuing voluntary credentials to individuals who have attained those qualifications. The Commission has adopted this *Code* to apply to individuals who hold these credentials.

The Ethics Code applies in its entirety to members of The American Dietetic Association who are Registered Dietitians (R.D.s) or Dietetic Technicians, Registered (D.T.R.s). Except for sections solely dealing with the credential, the *Code* applies to all American Dietetic Association members who are not R.D.s or D.T.R.s. Except for aspects solely dealing with membership, the *Code* applies to all R.D.s and D.T.R.s who are not ADA members. All of the aforementioned are referred to in the *Code* as "dietetic practitioners."

Principles

1. The dietetic practitioner provides professional services with objectivity and with respect for the unique needs and values of individuals.
2. The dietetic practitioner avoids discrimination against other individuals on the basis of race, creed, religion, sex, age, and national origin.
3. The dietetic practitioner fulfills professional commitments in good faith.
4. The dietetic practitioner conducts him/herself with honesty, integrity, and fairness.
5. The dietetic practitioner remains free of conflict of interest, while fulfilling the objectives and maintaining the integrity of the dietetic profession.
6. The dietetic practitioner maintains confidentiality of information.
7. The dietetic practitioner practices dietetics based on scientific principles and current information.
8. The dietetic practitioner assumes responsibility and accountability for personal competence in practice.
9. The dietetic practitioner recognizes and exercises professional judgment within the limits of his/her qualifications and seeks counsel or makes referrals as appropriate.
10. The dietetic practitioner provides sufficient information to enable clients to make their own informed decisions.

Figure 6.12
Code of Ethics for the Profession of Dietetics

11. The dietetic practitioner who wishes to inform the public and colleagues of his/her services does so by using factual information. The dietetic practitioner does not advertise in a false or misleading manner.

12. The dietetic practitioner promotes or endorses products in a manner that is neither false or misleading.

13. The dietetic practitioner permits use of his/her name for the purpose of certifying that dietetic services have been rendered only if he/she has provided or supervised the provision of those services.

14. The dietetic practitioner accurately presents professional qualifications and credentials.

    a. The dietetic practitioner uses "R.D." or "registered dietitian" and "D.T.R." or "dietetic technician, registered" only when registration is current and authorized by the Commission on Dietetic Registration.

    b. The dietetic practitioner provides accurate information and complies with all requirements of the Commission on Dietetic Registration program in which he/she is seeking initial or continued credentials from the Commission on Dietetic Registration.

    c. The dietetic practitioner is subject to disciplinary action for aiding another person in violating any Commission on Dietetic Registration requirements or aiding another person in representing himself/herself as an R.D. or D.T.R. when he/she is not.

15. The dietetic practitioner presents substantiated information and interprets controversial information without personal bias, recognizing that legitimate differences of opinion exist.

16. The dietetic practitioner makes all reasonable effort to avoid bias in any kind of professional evaluation. The dietetic practitioner provides objective evaluation of candidates for professional association membership, awards, scholarships, or job advancements.

17. The dietetic practitioner voluntarily withdraws from professional practice under the following circumstances:

    a. The dietetic practitioner has engaged in any substance abuse that could affect his/her practice.

    b. The dietetic practitioner has been adjudged by a court to be mentally incompetent.

    c. The dietetic practitioner has an emotional or mental disability that affects his/her practice in a manner that could harm the client.

18. The dietetic practitioner complies with all applicable laws and regulations concerning the profession. The dietetic practitioner is subject to disciplinary action under the following circumstances:

Figure 6.12
continued

a. The dietetic practitioner has been convicted of a crime under the laws of the United States which is a felony or a misdemeanor, an essential element of which is dishonesty and which is related to the practice of the profession.

b. The dietetic practitioner has been disciplined by a state, and at least one of the grounds for the discipline is the same or substantially equivalent to these principles.

c. The dietetic practitioner has committed an act of misfeasance or malfeasance which is directly related to the practice of the profession as determined by a court of competent jurisdiction, a licensing board, or an agency of a governmental body.

19. The dietetic practitioner accepts the obligation to protect society and the profession by upholding the *Code of Ethics for the Profession of Dietetics* and by reporting alleged violations of the *Code* through the defined review process of The American Dietetic Association and its credentialing agency, the Commission on Dietetic Registration.

Source: American Dietetic Association/Commission on Dietetic Registration. Code of Ethics for the profession of dietetics. *Journal of the American Dietetic Association,* 1999;99(1):109–113. Reprinted with permission. The Commission on Dietetics Registration. The American Dietetics Association, 1999.

Purpose of a Code of Ethics

The purpose of a professional code of ethics is to reflect the principles of the profession and to provide an outline of the obligations of the member of that profession to self, client, society, and the profession. The *Code of Ethics for the Profession of Dietetics* addresses the provision of professional services, the accurate presentation of credentials and qualifications, standards for avoiding conflict of interest, and accountability for professional competence in practice. The *Code* also speaks to compliance with laws and regulations concerning the profession, presentation of substantiated information, confidentiality of information, the honesty, integrity and fairness of the member, and the obligation to uphold the standards of the profession by reporting apparent violations.[7]

New members joining the ADA receive a copy of the code and sign a statement stating they will abide by it. A study conducted recently found that the majority of dietitians agree with and adhere to the *Code*.[8] The review process for violations of this code includes a review of the complaint, an investigation, a hearing, and, finally, a decision and recommendation. The alleged respondent may be acquitted or, if found guilty, censored, temporarily suspended, or expelled from membership.

COMMITMENT TO THE PROFESSION

Those demonstrating professionalism in dietetic practice have a sense of commitment to the growth of the profession, both as a field of intellectual endeavor and as a society where people of similar purpose band together.[9] This commitment is best demonstrated by active participation in a professional association. Professional associations rely heavily on the work of volunteers at all levels—local, state, and national (Figure 6.13). It is through this collective energy of many professionals working together that an association becomes dynamic and productive. As Peter Drucker has said, "No organization can do better than the people it has."[10]

The benefits of professional association membership are both tangible and intangible. The tangible benefits may include receipt of publications, continuing education opportunities, lobbying on key legislative

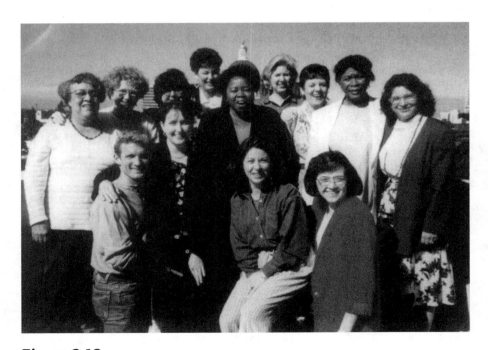

Figure 6.13
A state dietetic association executive board.

Source: California Dietetic Association. Reprinted with permission.

issues, public relations and marketing efforts, public recognition of professional achievements, student scholarship programs, member loan programs, discounts on rental cars and publications, travel programs, association-sponsored credit cards, group-rate medical and life insurance, and professional liability insurance, to mention just a few.

Of even greater importance are the intangible benefits that accrue from professional association involvement. The friendships that develop, the professional contacts that are made, the opportunity to develop leadership skills, the sense of creative stimulation, the excitement of being a part of the action, and the opportunity to impact issues and shape policy for the good of the profession are good reasons to volunteer at some level of commitment (Figures 6.14 and 6.15).

For students, there are additional advantages of active participation. Students have an opportunity to

- Develop skills in public speaking, writing, program planning, and organizing.
- Network with dietitians, technicians, and other students.
- Observe professional role models.

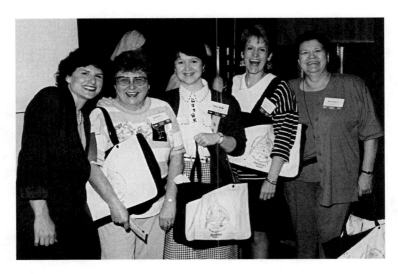

Figure 6.14
Camaraderie is shared among dietary managers at their annual meeting.

Source: Photo courtesy of the Dietary Managers Association.

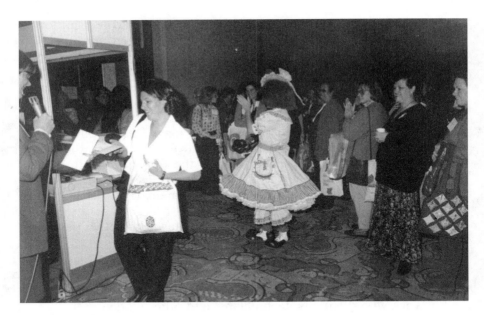

Figure 6.15
Dietitians enjoy some entertainment at their annual
meeting.

Source: California Dietetic Association. Reprinted with permission.

- Enhance visibility, for scholarships, internships, and future permanent employment.

The biggest risk one faces is the time commitment required. Frus-
trations may also arise when costs exceed the resources available for
certain plans or when members disagree. But these are minor considerations when one considers the risk of *not* being involved.[11]

SELECTED PROFESSIONAL ASSOCIATIONS

The American Dietetic Association

The nation's largest professional organization for food and nutrition
professionals, the ADA was founded in 1917 and now has approximately 69,000 members. There are a number of categories of membership with varying educational requirements for eligibility; however, the
majority of members are dietitians or dietetic technicians. Affiliated
dietetic associations exist in every state and in Puerto Rico and overseas. The mission of the ADA is to serve the public through the promo-

tion of optimal nutrition, health, and well-being. This association is discussed in more detail in Chapter 7.

The Dietary Managers Association

Founded in 1960, the Dietary Managers Association (DMA) is the national professional organization for dietary managers. Associate and student memberships are available. Total membership now exceeds 13,000. This association is discussed in more detail in Chapter 8.

American Institute of Nutrition

The American Institute of Nutrition (AIN) is the principal professional organization of nutrition research scientists in the United States. With approximately 3,000 members from 40 countries, AIN was chartered by the Regents of the University of the State of New York in 1933. To become a member, each person must be nominated by fellow scientists on the basis of demonstrated research competence and productivity in experimental nutrition or service to the discipline of nutrition. Graduate students who intend to pursue a career in nutrition research are eligible for membership. Those who have published meritorious original research in clinical nutrition are eligible for nomination for membership in the American Society for Clinical Nutrition (ASCN), the clinical division of AIN. ASCN publishes the *American Journal of Clinical Nutrition*. AIN is a corporate member of the Federation of American Societies of Experimental Biology (FASEB) and holds an annual meeting in conjunction with other FASEB societies. AIN publishes the monthly *Journal of Nutrition* and a quarterly newsletter, *Nutrition Notes*. AIN has an extensive awards and recognition program as well as a graduate research competition. It also publishes a graduate education directory.

American Society for Parenteral and Enteral Nutrition

The membership of the American Society for Parenteral and Enteral Nutrition (ASPEN) includes dietitians, nurses, physicians, pharmacists, and other healthcare providers involved or interested in nutrition support of patients. Student membership is also available. The organization publishes the *Journal of Parenteral and Enteral Nutrition* and *Nutrition in Clinical Practice* on a bimonthly basis; establishes and publishes standards and clinical guidelines for nutrition support; organizes and sponsors an annual multidisciplinary nutrition conference; administers a specialty certification program for nurses

PROFILE

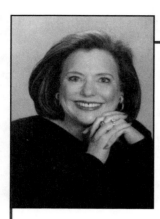

Mary Abbott Hess, L.H.D., R.D., L.D., F.A.D.A.

POSITION
   President, Hess & Hunt, Inc. Nutrition Commu-
      nications
   Evelyn Von Donk Steenbock Chair at the Uni-
      versity of Wisconsin-Stout
EDUCATION
   B.S. Simmons College, Boston, MA
   M.S. Northern Illinois University, DeKalb, IL
   L.H.D., Doctor of Humane Letters (honorary
      degree), Simmons College, Boston, MA
ROUTE TO REGISTRATION
   Dietetic internship

◆ Professional Involvement
   President, The American Dietetic Association, 1990–1991
   Chair, Food and Culinary Professionals Dietetics Practice Group
   Honors Committee member
   Charter Fellow of The American Dietetic Association
   Director-at-Large, ADA Board of Directors
   Board of Directors, American Dietetic Association Foundation
   Delegate from Illinois to ADA House of Delegates
   Member, International Association of Culinary Professionals
   Vice President of Chicago Chapter of Les Dames D'Escoffier

◆ Honors and Awards Received
   Evelyn Von Donk Steenbock Chair, University of Wisconsin-Stout profes-
      sorship to develop a state-of-the-art nutrition education and assess-
      ment center for the university
   First Place award for a text/reference book for *Portion Photos of Popular
      Foods*, Chicago Women in Publishing, 1998
   1998 Alumni of the Year, Northern Illinois University, DeKalb, IL
   First Place award for Books/Adult Trade for *The Art of Cooking for the
      Diabetic*, Chicago Women in Publishing, 1996
   1995 James Beard Award nominee for *The Healthy Gourmet Cookbook*
   Medallion Award, The American Dietetic Association, 1993
   President's Medallion, The American Culinary Federation, 1990
   Outstanding Dietitian of the Year, Chicago Dietetic Association

◆ Words of Wisdom for Future Dietetics Professionals

Food has power beyond its specific nutrients. In almost every area of dietetics practice, an understanding of food, how it should be prepared and served, and what eating it means to people, is essential. We must translate nutrition into food choices that meet the unique needs of each of our clients. Taking the time to care and share—asking the right questions and tailoring responses to individual (cultural, medical, social) needs makes each of us more effective as we communicate our expertise.

For most practitioners, continuing food education should be a life-long pursuit. Expand your own food horizons. If your food skills are limited, learn to cook. If you can't do it, you can't teach it! The emergence and phenomenal growth of the Food and Culinary Professionals dietetic practice group in the ADA demonstrates that many of the most successful members of our profession are seeking opportunities to enhance their food-related knowledge and skills. We must become the food experts we position our profession to be. As we learn more about the health benefits of specific foods (phytochemicals, nutraceuticals, etc.), we should merge this knowledge with food preparation techniques and encourage food choices that promote quality of life and health.

As dietitians, we often must work within limits of cost, fat, sodium, and so on. Like an artist who has 75 instead of 100 colors, we should help people eat beautifully and blend colors/foods that are available to create enjoyable meals and sustainable habits. We have learned from some past negative images of dietitians and foodservice that focusing on dietary restrictions (the missing 25 colors) makes us bad "artists" rather than creative ones. We need to work a bit harder to create great flavors that please the palate and to promote the pleasure of eating. Emphasize foods that are positive choices. This will reduce the need to talk about what should be restricted. Seek positive examples from chefs and food leaders, and look for opportunities to demonstrate your food expertise in your community. Use food to increase the power and quality of your practice!

and dietitians; provides a local chapter program; has awards and self-assessment programs; and serves as an advocate for nutrition support services.

Society of Nutrition Education

Members in the Society of Nutrition Education (SNE), both in the student and regular categories, are required to have at least two college-level courses in nutrition. The goal of the association is to enhance the ability of its members to help the public make informed food choices. Members are organized into practice divisions: communications, food and nutrition extension educators, higher education, international nutrition education, nutrition educators for children, nutrition educators with industry, public health nutrition, and sustainable food systems. A number of states have nutrition councils affiliated with SNE. The society publishes the *Journal of Nutrition Education* and the *SNE Communicator*.

National Restaurant Association

Founded in 1919, the mission of the National Restaurant Association (NRA) is to protect, promote, and educate the members of the foodservice industry. The NRA has 25,000 members representing more than 150,000 food-service operations. The benefits of membership include a monthly magazine, *Restaurants USA*; a weekly legislative report, *Washington Weekly*; research reports; educational seminars and materials; promotion of the industry to the government and the public; access to mailing lists and referrals; and annual shows. Membership is open to foodservice operators, businesses that provide products and services to the industry, students, and faculty. Dues are based on type of membership and annual gross sales of the business. Dietetic practitioners involved in foodservice management or sales and marketing of foodservice products find membership in NRA beneficial.

American Association of Family and Consumer Sciences

One of the oldest professional organizations in the field, the American Association of Family and Consumer Sciences (AAFCS) was founded in 1909 as a scientific and educational society and was then entitled the American Home Economics Association. Its founder, Ellen Richards, attended the Lake Placid Conference (see Chapter 1) and was instrumental in changing the name of the discipline from domestic science to home economics. The name of the organization was changed in 1994 to

AAFCS. Now, with nearly 20,000 members, its purpose is to improve the quality and standards of individual and family life through education, research, cooperative programs, and public information. Membership includes educators, lecturers, school administrators, extension home economists, counselors, child-care workers, dietitians, consultants, product development specialists, public relations directors, homemakers, and researchers. Each state has an affiliate association that sponsors meetings and programs throughout the year. The national association puts on an annual meeting and exposition.

National Association of Food Equipment Manufacturers

The active membership of the National Association of Food Equipment Manufacturers (NAFEM) is made up of commercial foodservice equipment and supplies manufacturers representing more than 600 companies in the United States and Canada. Industry trade publications are associate members of NAFEM. Founded in 1948, NAFEM's mission is to develop and promote cooperative programs and activities that will improve the level of professionalism and broaden knowledge within the foodservice equipment and supplies industry. Dietetic practitioners involved in layout and design consulting, and those in sales and marketing of foodservice equipment, find membership in NAFEM beneficial.

American School Food Service Association

The American School Food Service Association (ASFSA) was founded in 1946, the same year that the National School Lunch Act became law. Its mission is to protect and enhance children's health and well-being by operating nutritious foodservice programs and providing proper nutrition education in public and nonprofit private schools. Of more than 65,000 members, nearly 32,000 are certified through a program that requires the completion of coursework in sanitation, safety, technical skills, management, and nutrition. ASFSA publishes the *School Food Service and Nutrition Magazine*, a monthly trade journal, and the *Journal of Child Nutrition and Management*, a semiannual research journal. ASFSA has lobbied for legislation involving child nutrition policies and programs. The ASFSA sponsors a number of meetings and conferences throughout the year, including an annual conference and exhibition.

Foodservice Consultants Society International

Foodservice Consultants Society International (FCSI) has members in 30 countries. It publishes a quarterly journal, *The Consultant*; a member newsletter, *The Spec Sheet*; a membership directory; a products-buying guide; a bulletin, *FCSI/Tech*; and *Critical MAS*, a newsletter of case studies, opinions, and trends. To qualify for professional membership in FCSI, one must have at least ten years' experience as a foodservice consultant, four years of college, have been a project director for five years, be qualified to design and implement foodservice programs, be employed as a professional consultant, and submit an article of at least 2,000 words for publication in *The Consultant*. Other categories of membership, like student member, have less-strict requirements.

National Association of College and University Food Services

The mission of National Association of College and University Food Services (NACUFS) is to promote the highest quality of foodservice on school, college, and university campuses by providing educational and training opportunities, technical assistance, related industry information and support for research to the membership. The members of NACUFS are campus foodservice directors and support staff from over 540 colleges and universities in the United States, Canada, and abroad. NACUFS supports students with a summer internship program, scholarships, and awards. Benefits to members include networking opportunities from attending conferences, educational programs, and committee meetings; industry contacts; peer consultation services; educational and professional development programs; provision of comparative statistics; job placement; publications; professional recognition; and leadership opportunities.

SUMMARY

"A profession is shaped and molded by dynamic and dedicated individuals whose careers have made a difference."[12] The profession of dietetics requires a team approach with each member of the team the very embodiment of professionalism: knowledgeable, caring, concerned, respectful, ethical, committed to the profession, and active in the professional organization. The dietetic team member has an essential orientation to the interest of others—the patient, the client, the community, and others. The dietetic team member is unquestionably ethical in all matters. The dietetic team member is committed to preserving the credibility and dignity of the profession and believes that the practice of dietetics has an impact on the quality of life of others. Putting aside personal benefits and/or costs, the dietetic team member recognizes the importance of professional association involvement for the good of the profession as a whole.

SUGGESTED ACTIVITIES

1. Visit your school library to determine which nutrition periodicals are available. Carefully examine at least one issue of each, and write one or two sentences describing the journal. For example, one publication might be described as a monthly publication with literature reviews of nutrition research and occasional book reviews. Frequently, many articles in an issue are related to the same topic.

2. Carefully examine an issue of a popular magazine that contains articles on nutrition, such as *Shape* or *Hippocrates*. Briefly evaluate the reliability and validity of the nutrition content.

3. Attend a continuing education program sponsored by a local dietetic association. Write a report describing what is required of attendees to obtain continuing education credit.

4. Set some goals for professional development and self-improvement. Assign top priority to three, and describe why you chose these three.

5. Discuss the following scenario: A private practice dietitian regularly recommends that clients take megadoses of several vitamins. The dietitian bases the recommendation on years of research by a scientist who has testimonial evidence that the treatment works for a number of medical conditions. The dietitian's clients claim to have been helped when traditional medicine has failed. Has a code of ethics been violated? What are the issues here?

SELECTED RESOURCES

American Association of Family
   and Consumer Sciences
1555 King Street
Alexandria, VA 22314
703-706-4600 or FAX
   703-706-HOME

American Council on Science
   and Health
1995 Broadway,
   2nd Floor
New York, NY 10023-5860
212-362-7044

American Dietetic Association
216 West Jackson Blvd., Suite 800
Chicago, IL 60606-6995
312-899-0040

American Institute of Nutrition
   and The American Society for
   Clinical Nutrition, Inc.
9650 Rockville Pike
Bethesda, MD 20814-3998
AIN 301-530-7050
ASCN 301-530-7110 or
FAX 301-571-1892

American Medical Association
535 North Dearborn Street
Chicago, IL 60610
312-464-5000

American School Food Service
  Association
1600 Duke Street, 7th Floor
Alexandria, VA 22314-3436
800-877-8822 or FAX
  703-739-3915

American Society for Parenteral
  and Enteral Nutrition
8630 Fenton Street, Suite 412
Silver Spring, MD 20910
301-587-6315

Consumer Information Center
Pueblo, CO 81009

Dietary Managers Association
406 Surrey Woods Drive
St. Charles, IL 60174
800-323-1908 or 630-587-6336
  or FAX 630-587-6308
E-mail:
  http://www.dmaonline.org

Food and Nutrition Information
  Center
National Agricultural Library,
  Room 304
Beltsville, MD 20705
301-504-5719

Foodservice Consultants Society
  International
304 West Liberty Street, Suite 201
Louisville, KY 40202
502-583-3783

ILSI/The Nutrition Foundation
1126 Sixteenth Street, NW
Washington, DC 20036
202-857-3680

Institute of Food Technologists
221 North LaSalle Street
Chicago, IL 60601
312-782-8424

National Association of College
  and University Food Services
1405 South Harrison Road,
  Suite 303
Manly Miles Building, Michigan
  State University
East Lansing, MI 48824
517-332-2494 or FAX
  517-332-8144

National Association of Food
  Equipment Manufacturers
401 N. Michigan Avenue
Chicago, IL 60611-4267
312-644-6610 or FAX
  312-527-6658

The National Dairy Council
10255 West Higgins Road,
  Suite 900
Rosemont, IL 60018
847-803-2000

National Institutes of Health
9000 Rockville Pike
Bethesda, MD 20892
301-496-4000

National Restaurant Association
1200 Seventeenth Street, NW
Washington, DC 20036-3097
202-331-5900

Office of Disease Prevention and
  Health Promotion
National Health Information
  Center
P.O. Box 1133
Washington, DC 20013-1133
800-336-4797 or
  301-565-4167 (in Maryland)

Society for Nutrition Education
2001 Killebrew Drive, Suite 340
Minneapolis, MN 55425-1882
800-235-6690 or FAX
    612-854-7869

NOTES

1. Gove PB, ed. *Webster's Third New International Dictionary*. Springfield, Mass.: G & C Merriam Co., 1971.

2. Combs AW, Avila DL, Purkey WW. *Helping Relationships: Basic Concepts for the Helping Professions*. Boston: Allyn & Bacon, Inc., 1976.

3. Committee on Goals of Education for Dietetics, Dietetic Internship Council, The American Dietetic Association. Goals of lifetime education of the dietitian. *Journal of the American Dietetic Association*, 1969;54:91–93.

4. The American Dietetic Association Standards of Professional Practice for Dietetics Professionals. *Journal of the American Dietetic Association*, 1988;98:83–87.

5. Neville JN, Chernoff R. President's page: Professional ethics—everyone's issue. *Journal of the American Dietetic Association*, 1988;88:1285–1287.

6. American Dietetic Association/Commission on Dietetic Registration. Code of Ethics for the Profession of Dietetics. *Journal of the American Dietetic Association*, 1999;99(1):109–113.

7. *Ethics Resources*. Chicago, Ill.: American Dietetic Association, August 1986.

8. Anderson SL. Dietitians' practices and attitudes regarding the Code of Ethics for the Profession of Dietetics. *Journal of the American Dietetic Association*, 1993;93(1):88–91.

9. Mason M, Wenberg BG, Welsh PK. *The Dynamics of Clinical Dietetics*. 2nd ed. New York: John Wiley & Sons, Inc., 1982.

10. Drucker PF. *Managing the Nonprofit Organization*. New York: HarperCollins, 1990.

11. Dodd JL. President's page: The benefits and risks of membership. *Journal of the American Dietetic Association*, 1992;92:362.

12. Vickery CE, Cotugna N. *Legends and Legacies*. Dubuque, Ia.: Kendall/Hunt Publishing Co., 1990.

CHAPTER 7

The American Dietetic Association

The American Dietetic Association (ADA) is the largest association of nutrition professionals in the world.[1] Founded in Cleveland, Ohio, in 1917, the Association has grown to 69,637 members.[2,3] The purpose of this chapter is to help you understand the mission, vision, and values of the ADA and to become knowledgeable about the structure and organization of the ADA and its headquarters office.

WHO ARE THE MEMBERS OF ADA?

There are five classifications of membership in the ADA: active, associate, retired, returning student, and honorary.[4] You may use several of these membership categories as you move through your professional life.

Four types of individuals may apply for the active member classification. First, *active members* include any person who has a bachelor's degree from a regionally accredited college or university or its equivalent, meets academic requirements specified by ADA, and meets one or more of the following criteria:

1. Is a registered dietitian, credentialed by the Commission on Dietetic Registration.
2. Has completed a supervised practice program accredited/approved by the Commission on Accreditation/Approval for Dietetics Education (CAADE).
3. Has earned a master's or doctoral degree conferred by a regionally accredited college or university.

Second, any person may apply for active membership who has earned a master's or doctoral degree or equivalent, and who holds one degree (baccalaureate, master's, doctoral) in one of the following areas: dietetics, foods and nutrition, nutrition, community/public health nutrition, food science, or foodservice systems management. A regionally accredited college or university must confer each degree.

Third, any person who meets one or more of the following criteria may apply for active membership:

1. Is a dietetic technician, registered (D.T.R.) credentialed by the Commission on Dietetic Registration or has established eligibility to write the examination for dietetic technicians.
2. Has completed an associate degree program for dietetic technicians that has been accredited/approved by CAADE.
3. Is a graduate of a baccalaureate degree program and meets academic requirements specified by ADA, with CAADE-accredited or -approved dietetic technician program experience.

Finally, any person who has paid the optional one-time dues to obtain life membership in the ADA or has completed a term as president of the ADA may be an active member.

Associate members include any person who meets one of the following criteria and is not eligible for active membership:

1. Is a graduate of a baccalaureate degree program and meets requirements specified by ADA.
2. Is an undergraduate or associate degree student enrolled in a CAADE-accredited/approved dietetic program or is a graduate student meeting the minimum academic requirements in a CAADE-approved/accredited program.
3. Is a student enrolled in a supervised practice program accredited/approved by CAADE.
4. Is a student in a regionally accredited, postsecondary education program that is non-CAADE accredited/approved. This classification is available for three years to students who state intent to enter a CAADE-accredited/approved program.

See your dietetics program director for associate member information or call (800) 877-1600 for membership information. Joining ADA as a student is an excellent way to learn about the profession of dietetics and become familiar with its publications, activities, and other benefits.

Retired members include any member of ADA who is no longer employed in dietetic practice or education and is at least 62 years old or who is retired due to permanent disability.

The *returning student* category includes any active member returning to school on a full-time basis for a baccalaureate or graduate degree in a dietetic course of study. Membership in the returning student class can be held for a maximum of five years and must be renewed annually.

The *honorary member* category is a special honor awarded to an individual who has made a notable contribution to the field of nutrition and dietetics and has been invited to be an honorary member by the Board of Directors of the Association.

MISSION, VISION, PHILOSOPHY, AND VALUES

In the late 1980s, the ADA Board of Directors endorsed a mission statement that defines the purpose of the organization. The mission of the ADA is as follows:

> The American Dietetic Association is the advocate of the dietetics profession serving the public through the promotion of optimal nutrition, health, and well-being.[5]

The words *advocate, serving the public*, and *promotion* explain ADA's focus. The ADA acts as an advocate for its members, striving to position the dietitian as a nutrition expert in the eyes of the public, the medical community, legislators, and other constituencies. The members of the ADA serve the public in numerous ways, through the promotion of optimal nutrition and health.

The vision statement of the ADA serves as a guide to the officers of the ADA as they plan the programs and activities in which the organization will be involved. The vision statement helps members understand the role the ADA hopes to assume in the future. The vision statement of the ADA is as follows:

> Members of The American Dietetic Association will shape the food choices and impact the nutritional status of the public.[6]

The philosophy statement of the ADA sets the tone of customer service, which should be paramount in all interactions between dietitians and their clientele. The philosophy of the ADA states:

> Members of The American Dietetic Association serve the profession best by serving the public first.[7]

The values of the ADA serve as a guide to action and a statement of attributes toward which all dietitians should strive. The actions of the ADA and its members reflect the following values:

Excellence in the identification, development, and delivery of quality programs, services, and products.

Leadership in significant food, nutrition, and related health issues.

Integrity in all professional and personal actions.

Respect for diverse viewpoints and individual differences.

Communication that is timely and effective.

Collaboration for action on critical issues.

Fiscal responsibility in effectively providing and managing human and financial resources.

Action that is timely and strategic.[8]

ADA HEADQUARTERS

The headquarters of the ADA (216 W. Jackson Blvd., Chicago, IL 60606-6995, 800-877-1600) house the full-time paid staff members who carry on the day-to-day business of the ADA (Figure 7.1). Currently, the ADA has 151 paid employees.[9] Employees work in assigned groups that serve to support different aspects of ADA's focus.

Also located in Chicago are the American Dietetic Association Foundation, the National Center for Nutrition and Dietetics, and the offices of the Commission on Dietetic Registration (CDR).

The American Dietetic Association Foundation (ADAF) funds education initiatives that promote public nutrition, health, and well-being. The ADAF is considered to be a not-for-profit corporation and is the largest private grantor of scholarship and fellowship funds in the field of dietetics. Students in dietetics and related fields are encouraged to apply for ADAF scholarships. Applications are typically due the middle of February each year, with awards made for the following academic year. Dietetic education program directors receive information about these scholarships every fall.

The National Center for Nutrition and Dietetics (NCND) was established in 1990 as ADA's education center for the public. NCND contributes to ADA's mission of promoting optimal nutrition, health, and well-being through offering programs and services of interest to the public. These offerings include a toll-free Consumer Nutrition Hotline and R.D. referral service (800-366-1655), staffed by a registered dietitian. This hotline allows consumers to hear prerecorded nutrition messages, speak to a registered dietitian, and obtain referrals to R.D.s in their area. The NCND also sponsors National Nutrition Month, which is celebrated each March under the theme "Eat Right America" and Project LEAN (Low-fat Eating for America Now).

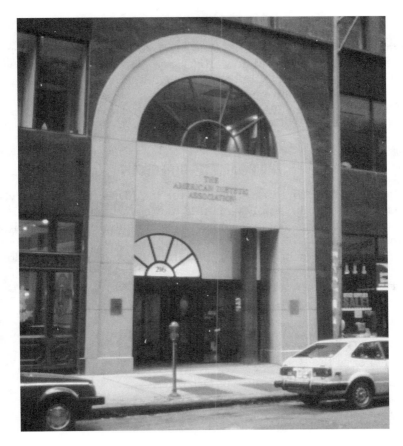

Figure 7.1
American Dietetic Association headquarters.

Source: Courtesy of American Dietetic Association.

The CDR is the credentialing arm of the ADA. The CDR credentials individuals who have met its standards for competency to practice in the profession. The function of CDR is more fully discussed in Chapter 5.

The ADA also retains paid employees at an office in Washington, D.C. (1225 Eye Street, N.W., Suite 1250, Washington, DC 20005). These employees work on ADA's behalf on legislative matters that affect the future of the dietetics profession. Members may call the ADA Office of Government and Legal Affairs in Washington at (202) 371-0500 if they have questions about legislative activities or issues affecting dietetics at the state or federal level.

THE VOLUNTEER ELEMENT OF ADA

The officers of the ADA are volunteers who are elected by the member-ship of the association. Major offices are elected by national ballot; members of particular subgroups elect officers of those subgroups (e.g., dietetic practice groups).

The work of the ADA is accomplished by two major entities: the Board of Directors and the House of Delegates.

THE BOARD OF DIRECTORS

The Board of Directors is responsible for the ADA's mission and vision and is the association's policy-making and governing body. The Board of Directors manages the property and fiscal affairs of the ADA, directs the implementation of approved actions, and monitors the outcomes of ADA projects. The board comprises the following elected positions:

President (Chairman of the Board of Directors)

President-Elect

Secretary/Treasurer

Secretary/Treasurer-Elect

Speaker of the House of Delegates

Speaker-Elect of the House of Delegates

President of the ADA Foundation

Chief Operating Officer

Five Directors-at-Large

Two Directors-at-Large Public Members (appointed by the Board of Directors)

Chair of the Commission on Dietetic Registration (no vote)

Chair of the Commission on Accreditation/Approval for Dietetics Education (no vote)

The two commissions that are represented on the Board of Directors are autonomous organizations, because of the nature of the business they conduct. These commissions direct accreditation of dietetic educa-tion programs and the credentialing of dietetics practitioners, two activi-ties that must remain free from the influence of the ADA. The Chairper-sons of these two commissions sit on the Board of Directors to facilitate communication between the commissions and the ADA; however, they do not vote on issues that are brought before the Board of Directors.

The Board of Directors uses several committees to accomplish its work. These committees include the Board of Directors Executive

Committee, the Budget and Fiscal Affairs Committee, the Legislative and Public Policy Committee, the Diversity Committee, and the Scholarship Committee.

THE HOUSE OF DELEGATES

The ADA House of Delegates is comparable to the U.S. House of Representatives. It provides a forum for membership and professional issues and establishes professional standards. Each state's dietetic association elects delegates to represent that state at the national level. The number of delegates a state has is based on the number of ADA members who live in that state. The House of Delegates has 138 members. The House of Delegates is divided into seven geographic areas, each with an Area Coordinator elected by national ballot. The Puerto Rico Dietetic Association has a representative in the House of Delegates, as does the American Overseas Dietetic Association, which represents American dietitians working abroad.

The ADA House of Delegates includes Area I with 18 delegates (Alaska 1, California 9, Hawaii 1, Idaho 1, Montana 1, Oregon 2, Washington 2 and Wyoming 1); Area II with 15 delegates (Iowa 2, Michigan 3, Minnesota 2, Missouri 2, Nebraska 1, North Dakota 1, South Dakota 1, and Wisconsin 3); Area III with 14 delegates (Alabama 2, Arkansas 1, Florida 4, Georgia 2, Louisiana 2, Mississippi 1, Puerto Rico 1, and South Carolina 1); Area IV with 16 delegates (Arizona 2, Colorado 2, Kansas 2, Nevada 1, New Mexico 1, Oklahoma 2, Texas 5, and Utah 1); Area V with 16 delegates (Illinois 4, Indiana 2, Kentucky 2, Ohio 5, Tennessee 2, and West Virginia 1); Area VI with 13 delegates (Delaware 1, District of Columbia 1, Maryland 2, North Carolina 2, Pennsylvania 5, and Virginia 2); and Area VII with 20 delegates (Connecticut 2, Maine 1, Massachusetts 3, New Hampshire 1, New Jersey 3, New York 7, Rhode Island 1, Vermont 1, and the American Overseas Dietetic Association 1).

The House of Delegates also includes the Speaker, who serves as the Chairperson; the Speaker-Elect; 7 Area Coordinators; 15 Delegates who make up the Council on Professional Issues (8 representing dietetics practice, 3 representing dietetics education, 3 representing dietetics research, and 1 Dietetic Technician-at-Large); and 2 other Dietetic Technicians-at-Large.

The full House of Delegates meets twice a year, immediately before the start of the annual meeting each fall and at the House of Delegates Mid-Year Meeting, typically held at the end of April or beginning of May. Issues are discussed and debated both in Area meetings and before the full House of Delegates. Since delegates are the elected representatives of ADA members in their respective states, they bring to these discussions the views of their constituents back home. Observers are welcome to attend any of these sessions to gain a fuller appreciation of how the work of the ADA is carried out. The formal House of Delegates meeting, during which agenda items are voted on, is held on Sunday each time the House of Delegates meets. It is a formal and impressive event.

STATE AFFILIATES AND DISTRICT DIETETIC ASSOCIATIONS

Each state and the District of Columbia has its own state dietetic association affiliated with the ADA. When individuals join the ADA, a percentage of their dues is rebated to the state dietetic association with which they wish to affiliate. While most individuals are members of the affiliate dietetic association of the state in which they live or work, a 1998 bylaws amendment now allows individuals the option to designate any state dietetic association for their membership. State dietetic associations elect their own officers and host their own meetings once or twice a year.

Each state association comprises district dietetic associations that serve the needs of dietitians in specific geographic areas within the state. There are currently approximately 220 district associations in the United States. District associations may comprise a single metropolitan area or several counties. Membership in district associations is *not* automatic. These groups receive no rebates from the national level and typically charge a separate membership fee to support their programming efforts.

Involvement in district and state dietetic associations is a great way for new dietetics graduates to become involved in a professional organization. Opportunities for leadership development and personal/professional growth abound in these groups.

DIETETIC PRACTICE GROUPS

Because of the increasingly specialized nature of dietetic practice, the leadership of ADA developed Dietetic Practice Groups (DPGs). DPGs comprise individuals who have a common interest in a particular area of dietetics practice, regardless of membership classification or employment status. A DPG may be formed when at least 300 members petition the House of Delegates Council on Professional Issues to form such a group.

DPGs are national in scope and have their own elected officers and dues. These groups engage in activities that meet the needs of their members, such as producing newsletters or providing continuing education events. These groups provide members the opportunity to

PROFILE

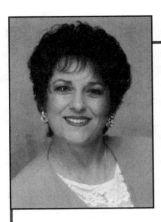

Penny Walters, D.T.R.

POSITION
> Springhouse Assisted Living, Boynton Beach, FL

EDUCATION
> A.A. Palm Beach Community College, Palm Beach, FL

◆ **Honors and Awards Received**
Florida Dietetic Technician of the Year
Excellence in Practice Award for Dietetic Technology from the American Dietetic Association Foundation

◆ **How Did You Find Out About Dietetics and Decide to Become a Dietetic Technician, Registered?**
In 1984, I enrolled in a computer technology course to retool for a new career. After just one semester, I realized that computer technology was *not* for me. While looking through the course catalog, *dietetics* jumped out at me—it was a blend of all things I held near and dear to my heart. Having done catering and bookkeeping most of my life, and having a keen interest in healthy eating, dietetics was right up my alley.

I changed my major and enrolled in the dietetic technician program at Palm Beach Community College. I completed my two clinical practica at local hospitals and my management practicum at a local nursing home. I graduated in May 1987 and became one of the first dietetic technicians to become registered by sitting for the credentialing exam.

After graduation, I decided to pursue a career in management and began my own consulting business. My clients included various adult congregate living facilities, weight loss programs, local hospitals needing vacation relief, a local "fat farm" that needed someone to oversee food preparation, and Palm Beach Community College, where I taught basic food preparation and nutrition classes. Having a consulting business allowed me time for involvement with my professional association as well.

In 1989, I founded a support group and a job bank for dietetic technicians in the Palm Beach area. This was a great support and networking opportunity, especially for new technicians coming into the area. In 1990 and again in 1993, I accepted positions in the foods and nutrition departments of hospitals and long-term care facilities in need of guidance and structure. In both instances, my education and training served me well, enabling me and the staff to reduce turnover, increase customer satisfaction, and come in under budget. I was able to ease back into clinical dietetic practice, learning about the new federal Medicare guidelines and other changes that had occurred in clinical practice.

My current position is regional director of foodservice systems for Springhouse Assisted Living. On any given day, long-term care residents interact with the foodservice department more than any other department in the facility. I work closely with the corporate dietitians, who provide assistance with menus, forms, and systems. It has been exciting to oversee the foodservice operations of the twelve Springhouse facilities, and our division continues to grow.

I have been very fortunate over the years to have support and assistance from many mentors. I have been able to perform my job duties as described and am very proud to say I'm a registered dietetic technician!

develop leadership skills through participation on committees or through appointment or election to offices. DPGs also provide a way for members of ADA to network within their area or areas of interest and practice. Figure 7.2 is a list of the current DPGs of the ADA.[10] Currently, there are 29 DPGs, and members of ADA may join as many DPGs as they desire. Dues are paid annually when ADA dues are paid. Dues vary from $10 to $25 a year.

DPG membership affords a member the following opportunities:

- Increase knowledge in a specific area of dietetic practice through newsletters, publications, and continuing education.
- Develop, sponsor, and/or attend workshops and seminars for continuing education credit at the ADA Annual Meeting and throughout the year.
- Develop legislative and public policy materials for ADA.
- Contribute technical expertise to ADA.
- Establish activities that market the profession in general and the practice area in particular.
- Provide guidelines for practice and quality assurance materials to help practitioners provide a high level of care.
- Provide support to individuals following a vegetarian lifestyle.[11]

Clinical Nutrition Management: Managers who direct clinical nutrition programs across the continuum of care.

Consultant Dietitians in Health Care Facilities: Practitioners typically employed under contract who provide nutrition consultation to acute and long-term facilities, home care companies, health care agencies, and the foodservice industry.

Diabetes Care and Education: Members involved in patient education, professional education, and research for the management of diabetes mellitus.

Dietetic Educators of Practitioners: Educators of students enrolled in Dietetic Technician Programs, Didactic Programs in Dietetics, Coordinated Programs in Dietetics, Approved Pre-Professional Practice Programs (AP4), Dietetic Internships, and other programs.

Dietetic Technicians in Practice: Dietetic technicians, dietetic technician educators, and dietetic technician employers who focus on the competencies, skills and needs of dietetic technicians.

Dietetics in Developmental and Psychiatric Disorders: Nutrition professionals whose work involves clients with physical and mental disabilities, developmental disorders, psychiatric illnesses, substance abuse problems and eating disorders.

Dietetics in Physical Medicine and Rehabilitation: Practitioners who provide nutrition support, counseling, and education to clients undergoing rehabilitation for inpatient/outpatient centers, group homes, transitional living centers, and industry.

Dietitians in Business and Communications: Professionals employed by, seeking employment in, or self-employed in the profit-making organizations of the food and nutrition industry.

Dietitians in General Clinical Practice: Practitioners who possess a mosaic of professional skills, provide and/or manage nutrition care in settings ranging from acute, to long-term, and maintain working knowledge in many clinical areas.

Dietitians in Nutrition Support: Practitioners integrating the science of enteral and parenteral nutrition to provide nutrition support to individuals in inpatient and outpatient settings, including transplantation, home care and pediatrics.

Environmental Nutrition: Members who are concerned with the environment and want to help improve modern dietary habits that affect our ecological balance.

Food and Culinary Professionals: Members who promote food education and culinary skills to enhance quality of life and health of the public.

Gerontological Nutritionists: Practitioners who provide and manage nutrition programs and services to older adults in a variety of settings—community, home health, health care facilities, and education/research facilities.

HIV/AIDS: Dietetics professionals sharing cutting edge information on nutrition management of HIV/AIDS. This practice group provides an avenue for research, monitoring, and advocacy for nutrition intervention.

Figure 7.2
The current DPGs of the American Dietetic Association.

Hunger and Malnutrition: Practitioners involved in local, national, and global promotion of adequate food and nutrition through advocacy, education, research, and legislation.

Management in Food and Nutrition Systems: Food and nutrition care managers generally employed in institutions, colleges, and universities; includes directors of departments or facilities and administrative dietitians and technicians.

Nutrition Education for the Public: Practitioners involved in the design, implementation, and evaluation of nutrition education programs for target populations.

Nutrition Educators of Health Professionals: Members involved in education and communication with physicians, nurses, dentists, and other health care professionals.

Nutrition Entrepreneurs: Consultants in the business of developing and delivering nutrition-related services and/or products. Membership ranges from veteran business owners to members establishing new practices.

Nutrition in Complementary Care: Dietetics professionals interested in the study of alternative and complementary therapies.

Oncology Nutrition: Nutrition professionals who are involved in the care of cancer patients, cancer prevention, and research.

Pediatric Nutrition: Practitioners who provide nutrition services for the pediatric population in a wide variety of settings including neonatal, nutrition support, cystic fibrosis, and WIC.

Perinatal Nutrition: Practitioners addressing nutrition care issues during preconception, pregnancy, postpartum, and lactation periods.

Public Health Nutrition: Local, state, and federal government nutrition professionals who work with all age groups in the public health arena.

Renal Dietitians: Practitioners who work in dialysis facilities, clinics, hospitals, and private practice renal nutrition counseling.

Research: Members who conduct research in the various areas of practice and are employed in the different practice settings of dietetics.

School Nutrition Services: Dietetic professionals engaged in the management of school foodservice and nutrition education programs at the local, state, or national levels or employed by companies providing products and services to these programs.

Sports, Cardiovascular, and Wellness Nutritionists: Nutrition professionals with expertise and skills in promoting the role of nutrition in physical performance, cardiovascular health, wellness, and disordered eating.

Vegetarian Nutrition: Nutrition professionals in community, clinical, education, or foodservice practice settings who wish to learn about plant-based diets and provide support to individuals following a vegetarian lifestyle.

Figure 7.2
continued

Source: American Dietetic Association. [www.eatright.org]. Reprinted with permission.

HONORS AND AWARDS BESTOWED BY THE
AMERICAN DIETETIC ASSOCIATION

Each year the ADA, ADAF, and DPGs honor individuals who have demonstrated outstanding contributions to the profession of dietetics. The *Marjorie Hulsizer Copher Award* is the highest honor the ADA can bestow on one of its members. Persons nominated for this honor must have contributed to the ADA through long, active participation and service. The recipient of this award is considered a trailblazer for the profession and someone who has contributed uniquely to the advancement of the profession. The Copher Award has been presented every year since 1945.

The *Lenna Frances Cooper Memorial Lecturer* presents a major paper related to his or her work in dietetics. The presentation of this lecture is a highlight of each Annual Meeting of the ADA. The topic presented is one of widespread interest to ADA members and is one normally associated with the lecturer's work. The recipient of this honor is a recognized speaker who has made noteworthy contributions to the profession of dietetics and who reflects the high standards and ideals personified by Miss Cooper, a pioneer in the ADA (Figure 7.3). A Cooper Lecturer has been recognized every year at the Annual Meeting of the ADA since 1962.

The *ADA Medallion* is awarded each year to a maximum of eight members of the ADA. The award is given in recognition of leadership, ability, and service. The first Medallions were given in 1976, and recipients of this award showcase the diversity of ADA members and their areas of practice.

Honorary membership in the ADA is one of the highest awards given to nonmembers. Each honorary member brings honor to the Association. Qualifications for nomination to honorary membership include distinguished contributions to dietetics through professional knowledge, technical expertise, and promotion of the ADA's mission, vision, and values; demonstration of goodwill through notable national or international service to the advancement of the profession and/or the Association; and promotion of dietetics professionals as contributors to the optimal health and nutritional status of the public. The first honorary membership was awarded in 1954.

The *ADAF Awards for Excellence in Practice* showcase individuals who have demonstrated exceptional performance in a practice area of dietetics through innovation and creativity in practice. Awards for excellence are given in Community Dietetics, Clinical Nutrition, Consultation and Private Practice, Management Practice, Education, Research, and Dietetic Technology.

The *Media Excellence Award* recognizes an individual who consistently reports nutrition information that is current, is scientifically

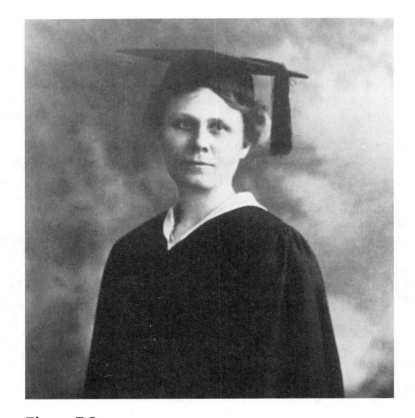

Figure 7.3
Lenna Frances Cooper, founding member.

Photo courtesy of The American Dietetic Association.

accurate, reaches a broad audience, is creative, and that positions dietetics professionals as experts in food and nutrition.

The *Presidents' Circle Nutrition Education Award* was created to recognize the development and dissemination of scientifically sound nutrition information that is unique in concept, creative in presentation, and free from specific commercial message or endorsement.

The *Anita Owen Award* encourages development of and recognizes excellence in innovative and unique models for delivery of food, nutrition, and dietetic information and/or innovative services for delivery of nutrition education to the public. This award recognizes the work of individual dietetics practitioners, not the specific program activities.

The *Judy Ford Stokes Award* is to encourage further development of administrative dietetics through cost-effective methods of revenue-generating techniques and/or foodservice facility design. The award is given to the person who submits the most creative cost study in either of these areas.

The *Huddleson Award* honors a registered dietitian who was the lead author of a peer-reviewed article that made an important contribution to the dietetics profession and that was published in the *Journal of The American Dietetic Association* during the previous calendar year.

The *Outstanding State Professional Recruitment Coordinator (SPRC) Award* recognizes dietetics professionals who have successfully developed, coordinated, and participated in their state affiliate's student recruitment network.

The *New Researcher's Award* recognizes the work of a new researcher in the field.

Distinguished Service Awards are bestowed on members of the U.S. Congress who have demonstrated outstanding service and support on nutrition and health issues of importance to the ADA and to the public.

The *Institutional Award for Excellence in Affirmative Action* recognizes the significant accomplishments of an ADA-accredited/approved dietetic education program in increasing and improving recruitment, selection, and support of ethnic minorities and male students.

The *Council on Practice, Dietetic Practice Group Awards* include the following:

- Gerontological Nutritionists DPG Joncier Greene Continuing Education Award
- Pediatric Nutrition DPG Published Research Award
- Pediatric Nutrition DPG Outstanding Member Award
- Pediatric Nutrition DPG Creative Nutrition Education Award
- Sports and Cardiovascular Nutritionist DPG Achievement Award
- Nutrition Research DPG Published Paper—First Author Award
- Nutrition Research DPG Published Paper—Contributing Author Award
- Nutrition Research DPG New Investigator Award

Among the honors and awards given by the affiliated state associations are these:

- Recognized Young Dietitians of the Year
- Recognized Dietetic Technicians of the Year
- Outstanding Dietetic Educators

- Outstanding Dietetic Students
- Outstanding Dietitian Awards
- Emerging Dietetics Leader Awards

WHY SHOULD I BE A MEMBER OF THE AMERICAN DIETETIC ASSOCIATION?

Membership in a professional association is a privilege. Professional associations like the ADA provide opportunities for personal and professional growth, leadership, and lasting friendships. Whereas one person alone may not feel that he or she can make a difference, the strength of almost 70,000 dietetics professionals can make their voices heard in setting public policy or influencing public opinion. The ADA plays a key role in influencing issues such as healthcare reform, food labeling, child nutrition programs, nutrition screening for the elderly, and long-term care. The ADA provides expert testimony at congressional hearings and comments on proposed federal and state legislation. The Association also publishes position papers, which outline ADA's stands on a variety of timely, and sometimes controversial, topics. ADA's homepage on the Internet (http://www.eatright.org) has an extensive listing of member services and benefits.

The ADA also conducts a number of important programs, campaigns, and other outreach efforts, to promote health and well-being and to position registered dietitians as nutrition experts. ADA's Strategic Framework for 1996–1999 outlines three major initiatives that provide direction for the work of the Association.[12] The first initiative is the Policy Initiative, which focuses on obtaining reimbursement for comprehensive nutrition services. The goal of this initiative is to convince policy makers at all levels of the value of comprehensive nutrition services and the contribution that these services make to maintaining a healthy population and to reducing the overall cost of healthcare. ADA is attempting to influence three key linkages. These are with the Federal government and its agencies, with state governments, and with the insurance industry, including managed care organizations.

The second major initiative of the ADA is the Member Initiative. The focus for this initiative is to enhance ADA members' ability to manage their careers, increase their skills, and learn how to apply those skills in unfamiliar environments. This initiative is particularly important because the work environment for many ADA members is changing rapidly due to dramatic changes in government policy, healthcare delivery systems, and other environmental changes. Several strategies to achieve this initiative include strengthening self-assessment skills of members, helping members acquire research and data management skills, assisting members in seeing how their skills can be transferred to other areas of dietetics practice or related fields, and training members in outcomes research.

The final initiative is the Public Initiative. The objective of this initiative is to influence the public's access to sound, scientifically based nutrition information and to increase ADA members' influence on consumers in the public debate concerning food and nutrition issues. Key linkages for this initiative include the public, policy makers, and the insurance industry, including managed care organizations. ADA members should be the preferred and most recognized source of consumer information on food and nutrition issues. Likewise, corporate and insurance industry demand for comprehensive nutrition services should increase, with dietetics professionals viewed as the leading provider of these services.[13]

SUMMARY

Belonging to the ADA, your state and district dietetic associations, and the ADA dietetic practice groups can enhance and enrich your professional and personal growth. Communication, networking, leadership opportunities, and other member benefits are available to those who participate. You determine your own level of involvement and, thus, your own level of satisfaction. Become actively involved in the ADA and reap the rewards of an active and involved professional life.

SUGGESTED ACTIVITIES

1. Attend a district, state, or national dietetics meeting.
2. Look for the issue of the *Journal of the ADA* that showcases the new officers of the ADA. Read the brief description about each person, and find out in what area of dietetics each person works.
3. Invite the delegate(s) to ADA's House of Delegates from your state to your class to talk about current issues relevant to dietetics.
4. Does your school have a Student Dietetic Association (SDA)? If so, do you actively participate? If not, attend the next meeting, and find out what is going on. If your school does not have an SDA, get together with your classmates and form such an association. Contact other schools that have dietetics programs to find out if they have an SDA and what types of activities they sponsor.

NOTES

1. The American Dietetic Association. *The American Dietetic Association: Promoting Better Health Through Better Nutrition.* Chicago, Ill.: The American Dietetic Association, 1995.

2. Cassell JA. *Carry the Flame: The History of The American Dietetic Association.* Chicago, Ill.: The American Dietetic Association, 1990.

3. The American Dietetic Association, Membership Committee. *House of Delegates Fall Meeting Report.* Chicago, Ill.: The American Dietetic Association, October 1998.

4. Bylaws of The American Dietetic Association. Amended by the House of Delegates, October 18, 1998, Kansas City, Mo.

5. Ibid.

6. Ibid.

7. Ibid.

8. Ibid.

9. The American Dietetic Association. *1998–1999 Directory of The American Dietetic Association* [On-line]. Chicago, Ill.: The American Dietetic Association, 1998. Available: http://www.eatright.org/dpg.html

10. Ibid.

11. The American Dietetic Association. *Dietetic Practice Groups.* Chicago, Ill.: The American Dietetic Association, 1998.

12. The American Dietetic Association. *The American Dietetic Association: Creating the Future. 1996-1999 Strategic Framework.* Chicago, Ill.: The American Dietetic Association, 1996.

13. Ibid.

CHAPTER 8

$\diamond$

The Dietary Managers Association

A brochure from the Dietary Managers Association states, "If you have enjoyed a hot lunch at school, been admitted to a hospital, or shared dinner with a family member or friend in a retirement community, chances are you had indirect contact with a professional dietary manager."[1] Who is the dietary manager?

The membership of the Dietary Managers Association (DMA) shows that dietetic management is a young profession on the move. Membership in the DMA has increased by more than 16,000 in just over 35 years.

Members of this association have been trained in foodservice operations management. In partnership with dietitians, they usually supervise and manage dietetic services in long-term care facilities, hospitals, schools, the military, correctional institutions, and other noncommercial foodservice operations.

The DMA promotes and maintains the competency of its members by making a certified credential available. The certified dietary manager must pass a competency exam and participate in a specified number of hours of continuing education. Like the ADA, the DMA has adopted a Code of Ethics to promote and maintain the highest standards of professional and personal conduct among its members. In addition, a wide array of benefits are available to members of the association.

FROM THE BEGINNING

In 1960, the Hospital, Institution, and Educational Food Service Society (HIEFSS) was founded and incorporated in the State of Illinois. The first meeting of HIEFSS was held in Cleveland, Ohio, and was attended by 72 prospective members from 15 different states. Representatives from The American Dietetic Association (ADA) were also present and participated actively in all decisions made at this meeting. The Board of Directors of the new association was established with five voting members. The Board was expanded to 15 voting members in 1978, as part of a reorganization of the association.[2]

The most common title used by members in 1960 was *foodservice supervisor*. In an effort to develop a career ladder of titles within the dietetics profession, the leadership of the ADA changed the title designation to *dietetic assistant* in 1971. A role delineation study was conducted by Ohio State University between 1981 and 1983. This study was underwritten by HIEFSS and the Certifying Board for Dietary Managers. As a result, the designated professional title was changed to *dietary manager*.

In July 1984, HIEFSS became the Dietary Managers Association. Following the establishment of the certifying board for dietary managers, the first credentialing examination was offered in 1985. In 1984, DMA and Purdue University entered into an agreement that established the Center for Professional Development. In 1985, Purdue granted continuing education credits to those attending educational sessions at the DMA annual meeting. Under the auspices of the Center, Purdue faculty develop and present Skill Builder Workshops designed around the ten areas of responsibility identified by the role delineation studies. A correspondence course on Professional Cooking was also developed and has been used by individuals in this country as well as in England, Australia, Italy, and Canada.

Membership in the DMA exceeded 16,000 in 1998; more than 70 percent of these members were certified.[3] Public relations activities, such as the dissemination of press releases, placement of commercial advertising, and promotions of free brochures, are a major part of the DMA's mission.

Although some facilities and educational programs continue to call trained individuals *foodservice supervisors*, the DMA works diligently to promote use of the title *dietary manager*. Currently, more than two-thirds of DMA members have been certified. One state requires that all dietary managers be certified; similar legislation is being considered by several other states.

To recognize the work of foodservice staff, DMA established Pride in Food Service Week in 1991. Each year, the DMA promotes this celebration through the sale of merchandise (e.g., posters, buttons, and T-shirts), and DMA brochures offer suggestions for other ways to celebrate.[4]

MEMBERSHIP CATEGORIES

The DMA has four categories of membership. Active membership in the association has always required the completion of a specific training program, including both classroom learning and supervised practice experience. **Active membership** is available to those who have graduated from a dietary managers training program approved by DMA. **Active certified membership** is offered to those individuals who have completed the DMA-approved training program, passed the credentialing exam, and applied for certification.[5]

Individuals who have completed an associate, bachelor's, or advanced degree in foodservice, healthcare, or a related field may become **associate members**. All membership benefits are available to Associate Members, except the right to vote or hold office. **Student membership** is open to those currently enrolled in a DMA-approved training program. Student members, too, are eligible for all benefits except voting privileges and holding office. Students are not eligible to take the credentialing exam until they have completed the training program.

THE CERTIFIED CREDENTIALS

C.D.M. (certified dietary manager) may be listed after a dietary manager's name when he or she has passed a competency exam administered by a testing firm and applied for certification through the Certifying Board for Dietary Managers. The Certifying Board is independent of DMA and comprised of six individuals—three members of DMA and three representatives of the allied professions, the general public, and employers of dietary managers.

Six categories of people are eligible to take the dietary managers credentialing exam: (1) active members of DMA; (2) nonmembers of DMA who have completed a DMA-approved dietary managers course; (3) nonmembers of DMA who hold a two- or four-year degree in foodservice management and nutrition; (4) associate members of DMA with a two- or four-year degree in foodservice management and nutrition; (5) associate members of DMA who have graduated from a state-approved or other accredited course and who have two years of experience (80 percent management/20 percent nutrition); and (6) current and former members of the U.S. military who have graduated from an approved military dietary manager training program and have attained the grade of E-5.

The certifying exam assesses competency in the areas of responsibility identified by the role delineation studies. The exam has been offered since 1985. The exam consists of 225 questions divided into two parts. Part I contains 150 questions, which cover ten competency areas under three major headings: nutrition, systems management, and administration/production management. In Part II, the remaining 75 questions specifically address foodservice safety and sanitation. Examinees must now pass both Part I and Part II of the exam to qualify for certification. Part II of the exam, which tests sanitation and food safety knowledge, was developed in 1996 to ensure that dietary managers are recognized as leaders in protecting public health.

Part I of the exam covers the following major content areas:

- Patient/Client Nutrition: Gather nutrition data; apply nutrition data.
- Patient/Client Service: Provide foodservices; provide nutrition education.
- Foodservice Personnel: Hire and supervise; develop personnel communications; interact with other professionals.
- Food/Kitchen: Manage supplies, equipment use, sanitation, and safety.
- Food/Service: Manage production.
- Financial: Manage business operations.

In Part II, the examinee must demonstrate knowledge in the following sanitation and safety content areas:

- Purchase, receive, and store food following established sanitation and quality standards.
- Protect food in all phases of preparation, holding, service, cooling, and transportation.
- Supervise foodservice personnel in the production and distribution of food in institutions.
- Select materials, equipment, and chemicals to ensure safety.
- Implement a food safety system that complies with regulations and Hazard Analysis Critical Control Point (HACCP) principles and recommendations from the Food and Drug Administration's new Model Food Code.

Passing the exam certifies that the individual is capable of competently performing the entry-level responsibilities expected of a professional dietary manager.

C.D.M.s work together with registered dietitians and registered dietetic technicians to provide quality nutritional care for patients/residents and perform the following tasks on a regular basis:

Interview patients/clients for diet history.

Conduct routine nutritional screening/assessment.

Calculate nutrient intake.

Identify nutrition problems and needs.

Implement diet plans and physicians' diet orders using appropriate modifications.

Use standard nutrition care procedures.

Document nutrition information in the medical record.

Participate in patient/client care conferences.

Counsel patients on basic diet restrictions.

Specify standards and procedures for food preparation.

Continuously improve care and service using quality management techniques.

Supervise preparation and serving of therapeutic diets and supplemental feedings.

Manage a sanitary foodservice environment.

Protect food in all phases of preparation, holding, service, cooling, and transportation.

Purchase, receive, and store food following established sanitation and quality standards.

Purchase, store, and ensure safe use of chemicals and cleaning agents.

Manage equipment use and maintenance.

Develop work schedules, prepare work assignments.

Prepare, plan, and conduct departmental meetings and in-service programs.

Interview, hire, and train employees.

Conduct employee performance evaluations.

Recommend salary and wage adjustment for employees.

Supervise, discipline, and terminate employees.

Supervise business operations of dietary department.

Write purchase specifications and orders for food, supplies, and equipment.

Develop annual budget, and operate within budget parameters.

Develop and implement policies and procedures.

To maintain the C.D.M. credential, an individual must earn 45 hours of continuing education credit every three years. This requirement ensures that the certified dietary manager remains up-to-date on the latest information in the field of dietary management.[6]

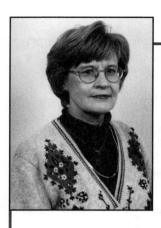

PROFILE

Helen Wiles, C.D.M.

POSITION
   Director of Food Service, Sisters of St. Joseph
      of Wichita, KS
EDUCATION
   Wichita Area Vocational-Technical College,
      Wichita, KS
ROUTE TO CERTIFICATION
   Dietary manager program through the Wichita
      Vocational-Technical College and work
      experience at Showalter Villa, Hesston, KS

◆ **How Did You First Hear About Dietetics and Decide to Become a Dietary Manager?**
In 1980, a friend who was working in a nursing home mentioned how much she had learned about nutrition in her position as a dietary aide. At the time, I had just closed a ceramic shop in Hesston, KS, and was looking for employment. I realized how much I enjoyed working in days past as a waitress, cook, and salad preparation person during high school. I enjoyed the idea of entering the field of nutrition, so I applied for the position at Showalter Villa. The administrator then asked me if I would consider going to the dietary managers course. I was thrilled to have the opportunity to go to school to learn more about nutrition.

◆ **Positions Held**
Various food management positions at Showalter Villa, Hesston, KS
Augusta Medical Complex, Augusta, KS
Prairie Homestead Retirement Center, Wichita, KS
Wichita Presbyterian Manor, Wichita, KS

◆ **Professional Involvement**
President, Wichita District Dietary Managers Association
President-Elect of Kansas Dietary Managers Association
Invited speaker for graduation ceremony for dietary managers at the
   Wichita Vocational-Technical College

◆ **Words of Wisdom for Future Dietetics Professionals**
Don't let go of your dreams! Always have short-term goals, along with long-term ones. Do what you enjoy in the dietetics field, and don't let anything come between you and what you enjoy. Be honest, fair, flexible, and positive. Always look for ways to improve what you are doing,

and keep an open mind. Stay involved with your professional association, and keep education offerings in mind when you are problem solv-
ing. Work in the field of dietetics is so rewarding because we are
allowed to serve our customers and improve their quality of their lives.

CERTIFIED FOOD PROTECTION PROFESSIONAL

Any foodservice professional may choose to take only Part II of the
exam, passage of which will allow an individual to use the certified
food protection professional (C.F.P.P.) credential with his or her name.
This credential is now recognized as the qualification for managing
food safety. To qualify to take this part of the exam, individuals who
are not already C.D.M.s must first complete DMAs new Food Protection Training Course or any other DMA-approved food safety and sanitation training curriculum. To maintain this credential, a C.F.P.P. must
complete five hours of continuing education relating to sanitation and
safety every three years.[7,8]

THE DMA CODE OF ETHICS

One of the requirements of a profession is that it regulate the ethical
conduct of its members. DMA promotes and maintains the highest
standards of professional and personal conduct among its members
through the adoption and enforcement of its code of ethics (Figure
8.1).[9] Adherence to the code is required for membership.

BENEFITS OF MEMBERSHIP IN DMA

The major emphasis of DMA is education and continuing education.
An annual meeting is held that includes exhibits and educational programs. District, state, and national meetings feature speakers on topics of relevance to the field. The Center for Professional Development
makes educational programs available across the country.

The Dietary Manager magazine is published bimonthly and sent
to all members. It includes nutrition and management feature articles,
product information, legislative news, book reviews, classified advertising, tips for professional development, and professional association
information. Several reference books are produced by DMA and
offered to members at reduced prices.

As a member of Dietary Managers Association, I pledge myself to:

- Reflect my pride in my competence as a dietary manager by wearing my pin and emblem and displaying my certificate.
- Use only legal and ethical means in the practice of my profession.
- Use every opportunity to improve public understanding of the role of the dietary manager.
- Promote and encourage the highest level of ethics within the industry.
- Refuse to engage in, or countenance, activities for personal gain at the expense of my employer, the industry, or the profession.
- Maintain the confidentiality of privileged information entrusted or known to me by virtue of my position.
- Maintain loyalty to my employers, and pursue their objectives in ways that are consistent with the public interest.
- Always communicate the administrative decisions of my employer in a truthful and accurate manner.
- Communicate to proper authorities, but disclose to no one else, any evidence of infraction of established rules and regulations.
- Strive for excellence in all aspects of management and nutritional practices, with constant attention to self-improvement.
- Maintain the highest standard of personal conduct.

Figure 8.1
The Dietary Managers Association code of ethics

Source: Dietary Managers Association. *Code of Ethics*. St. Charles, Ill.:
Dietary Managers Association. Courtesy of Dietary Managers
Association.

DMA is headquartered in Illinois; it has a Washington, D.C., office to monitor and impact legislation affecting dietary managers. At the grassroots level, volunteer efforts like letter-writing campaigns are used to influence pending healthcare reform legislation.

Participation on a local level offers members education, camaraderie, peer support, and opportunities for networking. Holding an office in DMA offers personal and professional gratification and the opportunity to further develop leadership abilities.

The DMA employment exchange program is available free to members and confidentially matches job seekers with a computer-generated listing of job openings in the desired locale. This computer database is maintained by the membership services department and may be used by job seekers and those who have employment opportunities.

DMA encourages members to call its toll-free number (800-323-1908) for answers to their questions regarding current trends, education opportunities, association activities, and any other areas of need. Members receive a certificate of membership suitable for framing and a plastic membership card. Optional benefits include group-rate insurance programs, a VISA card with the association's logo on it, and special car rental rates.

SUMMARY

DMA's slogan says it all: "The Dietary Managers Association is an organization of professionals dedicated to achieving excellence in the food service industry." This relatively young professional association sets high ideals for itself and its members. Standards of professional and personal conduct have been carefully written and communicated to the membership. The standards are measurable and attainable and serve to define the profession.

Membership is limited to those who have met the requisite educational standards, which include both academic learning and hands-on experience in approved programs. Those who aspire to an advanced level of professional status may demonstrate their competence by successfully completing a credentialing exam.

The primary focus of DMA is educational. Opportunities are provided for member education via publications, meetings, exhibits, a bimonthly magazine, workshops, and courses. DMA also provides members with peer support, professional recognition, public relations for the profession, opportunities for networking, career guidance, legislative representation, and other valuable benefits.

SUGGESTED ACTIVITIES

1. Locate a dietary manager in your area and interview him or her. A local community college or technical school that offers the DMA-approved training course would be a good resource.

2. Compare and contrast the certified dietary manager credential to that of the registered dietitian. How are they alike, and how do they differ?

3. A strong working relationship exists between the dietitian and the dietary manager. Describe why this is the case and how this relationship manifests itself.

NOTES

1. Dietary Managers Association. *Answers to your questions about dietary managers*. St. Charles, Ill.: Dietary Managers Association.

2. Dietary Managers Association. *History of Dietary Managers Association*. Itasca, Ill.: Dietary Managers Association, 1985.

3. St. John W. A look at the year ahead for DMA. *Dietary Manager*, 1994;3:32.

4. Dietary Managers Association. Tips for celebrating Pride in Food Service Week. *Dietary Manager*, 1993;2:27–29.

5. Dietary Managers Association. *Invest in Your Professional Success With Dietary Managers Association*. St. Charles, Ill.: Dietary Managers Association.

6. Dietary Managers Association. *CBDM Credentialing Exam*. St. Charles, Ill.: Dietary Managers Association.

7. Dietary Managers Association. *Earn the CFPP (Certified Food Protection Professional) Credential*. St. Charles, Ill.: Dietary Managers Association.

8. Dietary Managers Association. *Foodborne Illness . . . A Major Public Health Issue: DMA Provides the Solution*. St. Charles, Ill.: Dietary Managers Association.

9. Dietary Managers Association. *Code of Ethics*. St. Charles, Ill.: Dietary Managers Association.

PART FIVE

The Future

CHAPTER 9

Trends and Predictions

If we had a crystal ball and could look into the future, what would we see for the future of dietetics? What roles will dietitians play? What areas of practice that are unheard of now will exist in the twenty-first century? What will be the impact of technology on the practice of dietetics? Will the future needs of our clients be different from their needs today?

IDENTIFICATION OF TRENDS

One of the stated functions for ADA's House of Delegates is "identify and prioritize trends to guide the Board of Directors in developing strategic direction."[1] Each year, the House of Delegates members interview individuals and conduct research to determine these trends that will impact the future of the profession of dietetics. The cycle that is followed begins in the spring with the initiation of trends and issues data gathering. The Council on Professional Issues and the dietetics practice groups validate the trends. Throughout the summer months, delegates share information on trends and gather further data to validate the trends. In the fall, the identified trends are presented as formal input to the Board of Directors. During the winter, the Board of Directors, using the trend data, formulates the agenda of work for the upcoming year and develops the budget to carry out those plans. The following trends came from the 1998 House of Delegates and were reported at the Annual Meeting in Kansas City in October 1998. The trends are categorized by environment as social issues, technological issues, economic issues, and political issues. Trends are also identified in relation to the major practice areas in dietetics such as clinical issues; community issues; food and nutrition management issues; and research, education, and credentialing issues. Last, consumerism issues are addressed.

Social Issues

- Consumer access to health improvement resources is being limited by healthcare plans.
- The population is aging.
- Consumers' use of complementary therapies is increasing.
- Consumers are demanding convenience in products and services.
- Consumers are demanding faster information and faster results.
- Employer-granted time for professional education and volunteering is decreasing.
- The need for professional networking is increasing.

Technological Issues

- Technology use (computers, videos, fax, lasers, satellites, online services and e-mail) is on the rise.
- Consumers are using technology more to interactively access information.
- The rate of technological research and development and the need for management of information is increasing.
- Computer-driven information products are being substituted for patient interaction with dietetics professionals for nutrition education.
- Use of technology in management, marketing, and new product development is increasing.
- New biotechnologies are rapidly being developed.

Economic Issues

- Insurance companies are increasingly reimbursing physicians and other nondietetics professionals for nutrition services.
- Salary scales for other health professionals are rising more rapidly than for those of dietetics professionals.
- More dietetics professionals are entering nontraditional employment.
- Full-time permanent employees are being replaced with contract employees, outside consultants, and independent operators.
- Independent entrepreneurial business opportunities are increasing.

- Membership in professional organizations is decreasing due to limited economic resources of individuals.
- Mid-level management is shrinking in number, increasing the responsibilities of direct providers.

Political Issues

- The Health Care Financing Administration (HCFA) is revising conditions of participation for hospitals, long-term care, and home healthcare with potential for impact on the delivery of dietetics services.
- Reimbursement to healthcare facilities is being reduced by the Federal government.
- Teaching hospitals can no longer stand up to the financial pressures being driven by managed care.
- Legislatures continue to view expansion of professional licensure with skepticism.
- There is a shift from reimbursement of practitioners to reimbursement for services provided.
- Licensure is moving from state licensure to regional licensure.

Clinical Issues

- Healthcare systems are placing increased emphasis on accountability and cost-effective outcomes.
- The continuum of care is shifting to integrative acute care, long-term care, home care, and community support.
- As hospitals are downsizing and outsourcing, opportunities for dietitians are shifting to new settings.
- Consumer use of complementary medicine modalities is increasing.
- The need to "do more with less" is increasing in healthcare facilities.
- The point of care is shifting from acute care to primary outpatient care.
- The blurring of discipline-specific job responsibilities is increasing.

Community Issues

- The number of meals prepared and/or eaten away from home is increasing.
- Media influence on consumer nutrition information is increasing.

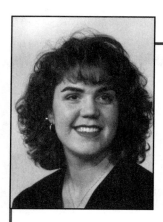

PROFILE

Lisa Friesen

POSITION
   December 1998, graduate in dietetics
EDUCATION
   Kansas State University, Manhattan, KS
ROUTE TO CERTIFICATION
   Coordinated Program in Dietetics

◆ **How Did You First Hear About Dietetics?**
Dietetics has always been a part of my life. I will be the third generation of dietitians in my family. My grandmother practiced administrative and clinical dietetics in a hospital, and my mother is a dietitian in a diabetes treatment center. I have been a lifelong student of these practicing dietitians, and with my interest in both science and working with people, it was a natural career choice.

◆ **What Are Your Professional Goals?**
My future professional goals are to practice clinical dietetics in an acute care facility, obtain a Ph.D. in nutrition, and speak, travel, and publish with the aim to educate other professionals and the public on the value of good nutrition. I am particularly interested in finding ways to use the Internet and telecommunications to make sound nutrition counseling available to people who have difficulty obtaining it in traditional ways. I have already helped develop some state-of-the-art web-based nutrition courses at Kansas State University, and I think this could be adapted into a useful medium for reaching the general public as well.

◆ **What Excites You About the Future of Dietetics?**
Increasing recognition of the value of good nutrition excites me. Researchers continue to discover and confirm the role nutrition plays in health, quality of life, and disease prevention. Dietitians are uniquely equipped with expertise in science-based nutrition, which gives us the privilege of helping the public and other professionals develop and evaluate new strategies for achieving optimal nutrition. Advancing technology presents an exciting new vehicle for dietetic information gathering and education as well. I look forward to using scientific and technological advances to meet the nutrition needs of all generations as conveniently and practically as possible.

◆ **What Advice Do You Have for Students Considering Dietetics as a Career Choice?**

My first piece of advice to students who are considering dietetics as a profession is to work hard to achieve and keep current the knowledge that makes you the nutrition expert. Knowing the science behind nutrition claims and strategies is crucial to separating nutritional truth from fiction and maintaining our professional credibility. Second, explore the nontraditional facets of dietetics. Versatility and keeping up with technological trends are vital for marketing yourself and our profession in an increasingly global and competitive world.

- Composition of foods is changing (use of fat substitutes, etc.).
- Community interest in health foods is increasing.
- Public awareness of food safety issues is rising.
- Health food and supplement suppliers are moving into the retail food market.
- Food security continues to grow as a national issue.

Food and Nutrition Management Issues
- Fast-food companies are replacing traditional school foodservice at all grade levels in many schools.
- Changing reimbursement systems are increasingly forcing facilities to reduce foodservice costs.
- Foodservice is increasingly being contracted out to management companies.
- Foodservice continues to be a growth industry, offering more career opportunities for dietetics professionals.
- Home delivery of groceries and ready-to-eat foods is increasing.
- Microwaved food consumption is increasing.

Research, Education, and Credentialing Issues
- Cross training of allied health professionals is increasing.
- The food and nutrition knowledge base is rapidly changing.
- Availability of healthcare time for student educational supervision is decreasing.
- There is a continued emphasis on lifelong learning to remain competitive in practice.

- The proliferation of credentials is making it more difficult to distinguish between providers of comprehensive nutrition services (R.D.s, nutritionists, etc.).
- Competency-based education continues to increase.
- Interest in food and nutrition-related careers is increasing.
- Use of communications technology for delivery of educational programs is increasing.

Consumerism Issues

- Members of non-science-based groups and others without appropriate food and nutrition training are aggressively positioning themselves as experts with the media.
- Consumer confusion regarding food and nutrition issues has increased.
- Consumer use of nutritional supplements has increased.
- Food and nutrition information (both accurate and inaccurate) is more readily available to consumers.
- Medical professionals not trained in nutrition, nutrition amateurs (e.g., models, movie stars, and others without proper credentials) are aggressively positioning themselves with the media as experts on food and nutrition topics.
- Consumers are increasingly using the Internet for information.
- Reporters at highly specialized media outlets are increasingly viewing and positioning themselves as experts and are not relying on credible, third-party advice.
- Consumers are assuming increased responsibility for their own health.

Reading through these lists of trends shows both the threats and opportunities facing the profession of dietetics and dietetics professionals in the coming years. The changes cited mean that dietetics professionals must be better informed, more computer literate, more entrepreneurial, and more aggressive in marketing themselves and their skills and abilities than ever before.

RESPONSES TO IDENTIFIED TRENDS

The House of Delegates summarized the recommended action for the ADA in responding to these trends:

ADA's Public Initiative
- Incorporate food security as an ADA initiative.
- Promote the dietetics professional as the preferred source of nutrition information.
- Focus on collaboration and alliance development.

Research
- Expand outcomes research and practice guidelines development.
- Educate ADA members to conduct research on staffing needs based on outcomes, acuity, and population.

Policy
- Develop alliances with third-party payers (insurance companies) to encourage preventive care.
- Provide skill-building opportunities for ADA members to learn how to work more effectively with federal agencies, regulatory bodies, and governmental processes.

Commission on Dietetic Registration
- Use the professional development portfolio system for career mentoring.
- Showcase ADA members who have learned new skills and moved into nontraditional roles.

Commission on Accreditation/Approval for Dietetics Education
- Shift education requirements to include more business skills, operations management and research, culinary skills, bilingual and cultural competencies, and cross training/upskilling.
- Increase opportunities for dietetics students to interact with professionals in case management, food science, the food industry, and complementary/alternative care.

Dietetics Practice Groups
- Conduct seminars for members.
- Develop "tool kits" for members.
- Provide mentoring programs.
- Conduct activities with students.

- Support food security issues.
- Provide information on complementary/alternative care.
- Promote food safety issues.
- Partner with food and foodservice industries.
- Provide training on business and communications skills.
- Identify emerging job areas and opportunities.

Foodservice
- Establish liaisons with the fast-food industry, restaurants, and schools.
- Expand recruitment and entry-level education in areas of foodservice management.
- Conduct advanced-level seminars on foodservice topics.
- Initiate a marketing campaign to position dietetics professionals in new foodservice markets.

Overall Continuing Education Needs
- Educate ADA members on career management and retooling, negotiation skills, nontraditional roles, entrepreneurial skills, marketing, and outcomes.
- Support professional development portfolio implementation by members through mentoring and providing learning resources.
- Provide a secure Web site for all members to assess their needs, skills, and career aspirations and receive tailored feedback on ADA benefits to the particular individual.[2]

SUMMARY

The future of dietetics is dynamic and exciting. Entrepreneurial dietitians, who see change as opportunity, will be the ones who take dietetics into the twenty-first century. Dietitians must be willing to seize opportunities to market themselves and their abilities in new and exciting ways.

According to Sara Parks, former ADA president, we must develop new consumer-responsive products and services, such as new foods, new approaches to nutrition education, new computer software, and new programs targeted at children, families, minorities, women, the elderly, and dual-career families. New areas of dietetic practice will be developed as new customer needs are discovered.[3]

The profession of dietetics has a bright and exciting future. Only your energy level and imagination will limit you. Prepare now to be a part of that bright future!

SUGGESTED ACTIVITIES

1. Review copies of the *Journal of the American Dietetic Association* and the *ADA Courier* for the past year. What hot topics are being discussed in these publications? How much do you know about these topics? How do you think these topics may affect your future practice in dietetics?

2. Read current issues of popular newspapers or news magazines, such as *The Wall Street Journal, Time, Newsweek,* or *U.S. News and World Report.* Look specifically for articles that might relate to dietetic practice, including health-related topics, food, nutrition, foodservice, public health, and so on. What implications might these topics have for dietetics?

3. Review the "President's Page" in each issue of the *Journal of the American Dietetic Association.* What topics have been discussed? What issues are facing the profession of dietetics or The American Dietetic Association?

NOTES

1. The American Dietetic Association. *House of Delegates Manual—1998–1999.* Chicago, Ill.: The American Dietetic Association, April 1998.

2. The American Dietetic Association. *American Dietetic Association House of Delegates Report,* personal communication, October 1998.

3. Parks SC. President's page: Challenging the future. *Journal of the American Dietetic Association,* 1994;94:89.

Index

Nightingale, Florence, 5
Nowlin, Bettye, 33
Nuclear medicine technologists, 51
Nursing, 49

Occupational therapists, 51
Outstanding State Professional
    Recruitment Coordinator
    Award, 145
Owen, Anita, 144

Pennsylvania Hospital, 4
Pharmacists, 49
Philadelphia Cooking School, 5–6
Philadelphia General Hospital, 4
Physical therapists, 50
Physician assistants, 51
Physicians, 47
  cardiology, 47
  endocrinology, 48
  neurology, 48
  oncology, 48
  ophthalmology, 48
  osteopathy, 48
  pathology, 48
  podiatry, 48
  psychiatry, 48
  surgery, 48
Practice, Standards of, 109,
    111–114
  continued competence and
    professional accountability,
    114
  knowledge, communication and
    application, 112
  quality in practice, 113
  research, application of, 111
  resources, utilization and
    management, 112
  services, provision of, 111
Presidents' Circle Nutrition
    Education Award, 144
Profession, 30
Professional association
    membership, 118–126
  American Association of Family
    and Consumer Sciences,
    124–125

American Dietetic Association,
    120
American Institute of Nutrition,
    121
American School Food Service
    Association, 125
American Society for Clinical
    Nutrition, 121
American Society for Parenteral
    and Enteral Nutrition, 121
benefits of, 118–119
Dietary Managers Association, 121
Federation of American Societies
    of Experimental Biology, 121
Foodservice Consultants Society
    International, 125–126
National Association of College
    and University Food Services,
    126
National Association of Food
    Equipment Manufacturers,
    125
National Restaurant Association,
    124
Society of Nutrition Education,
    124
Professional development, 91–92
Professionalism, 101–129
  commitment to, 118
  ethics of, 110, 115–118
  helping profession, 101
  professional associations,
    120–126
  standards of, 109, 111–114

Radiologic technologists, 51
Respiratory therapists, 51
Rorer, Sarah Tyson, 5–6

Senate Select Committee on
    Nutrition and Human Needs,
    13
Social Security Act, Title V, 11
Social workers
Society of Nutrition Education, 124
Soyer, Alexis, 5
Specialty areas, 30, 31–32
St. Bartholomew's Hospital, 3

DATE DUE

SEP 2 5 2006			